Sports Massage for Injury Care

Robert E. McAtee
LMT, BCMTB, CSCS

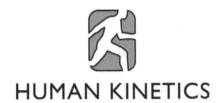

HUMAN KINETICS

Library of Congress Cataloging-in-Publication Data

Names: McAtee, Robert E., 1948- author.
Title: Sports massage for injury care / Robert E. McAtee, LMT, BCMTB, CSCS.
Description: Champaign : Human Kinetics, [2019] | Includes bibliographical
  references and index.
Identifiers: LCCN 2018043584 (print) | LCCN 2018044772 (ebook) | ISBN
  9781492588757 (epub) | ISBN 9781492560647 (PDF) | ISBN 9781492560630
  (print)
Subjects: LCSH: Sports massage. | Wounds and injuries. | Sports medicine.
Classification: LCC RC1226 (ebook) | LCC RC1226 .M33 2019 (print) | DDC
  615.8/22088796--dc23
LC record available at https://lccn.loc.gov/2018043584

ISBN: 978-1-4925-6063-0 (print)

This publication is written and published to provide accurate and authoritative information relevant to the subject matter presented. It is published and sold with the understanding that the author and publisher are not engaged in rendering legal, medical, or other professional services by reason of their authorship or publication of this work. If medical or other expert assistance is required, the services of a competent professional person should be sought.

The web addresses cited in this text were current as of December 2018, unless otherwise noted.

Senior Acquisitions Editor: Michelle Maloney
Developmental Editor: Laura Pulliam
Managing Editor: Dominique J. Moore
Copyeditor: Annette Pierce
Indexer: Nan N. Badgett
Permissions Manager: Martha Gullo
Graphic Designer: Denise Lowry
Cover Designer: Keri Evans
Cover Design Associate: Susan Rothermel Allen
Photograph (cover): © Human Kinetics
Photographs (interior): Jason Allen/© Human Kinetics
Photo Asset Manager: Laura Fitch
Photo Production Coordinator: Amy M. Rose
Photo Production Manager: Jason Allen
Senior Art Manager: Kelly Hendren
Illustrations: © Human Kinetics, unless otherwise noted
Printer: Walsworth

Human Kinetics books are available at special discounts for bulk purchase. Special editions or book excerpts can also be created to specification. For details, contact the Special Sales Manager at Human Kinetics.

Printed in the United States of America   10 9 8 7 6 5 4 3 2 1

The paper in this book was manufactured using responsible forestry methods.

Human Kinetics
P.O. Box 5076
Champaign, IL 61825-5076
Website: www.HumanKinetics.com

In the United States, email info@hkusa.com or call 800-747-4457.
In Canada, email info@hkcanada.com.
In the United Kingdom/Europe, email hk@hkeurope.com.

For information about Human Kinetics' coverage in other areas of the world,
please visit our website: **www.HumanKinetics.com**

This book is dedicated to the late John Harris, mentor, colleague, and friend. His teaching, writing, and friendship had a profound influence on me and set the trajectory for my career path as a sports therapist, writer, and teacher.

CONTENTS

PREFACE

Although many entry-level massage therapy training programs include 20 to 50 hours of event-oriented sports massage, the opportunities to acquire advanced, clinically oriented sports massage skills are difficult to come by. This book brings together in one resource a range of assessment and manual treatment techniques that are otherwise only found scattered throughout a variety of other books, journals, articles, blogs, and online videos.

Massage therapists have the ability to work with acute and chronic soft tissue injuries in a way that few other practitioners do. Massage practitioners occupy a special niche in the health care delivery system, as evidenced by the common and ongoing reports by clients and prospective clients that their conditions are not severe enough for them to consult their physicians but are interfering with their quality of life, their ability to pursue their athletic endeavors, or their ability to perform daily activities.

Physicians are generally limited to medication or surgery in their approach to treatment. Although the physical therapy profession is moving in the direction of manual therapy applications, many physical therapy clinics still rely heavily on treatment modalities such as ice, heat, dry needling, electrical muscle stimulation, and exercise to address soft tissue problems. These approaches can be effective and many times constitute an important component in the treatment of soft tissue trauma. Clinically oriented sports massage therapy is often the missing component in injury-rehabilitation programs.

When practicing clinically oriented sports massage, practitioners must be able to accurately evaluate and correctly treat the soft tissue injury, whether it be acute or chronic. Treating the injury without determining and helping to remedy its underlying cause leaves the athlete susceptible to reinjury. Clinical sports massage therapists must have broad knowledge in many areas, including biomechanics, proper training techniques for a variety of sports, strength training, diet and nutrition, and the myriad details related to specific sports and how they affect the body. This knowledge must then be applied as appropriate to help their athletes recover from injuries and prevent their recurrence.

This book covers many of the most common soft tissue sports injuries, their causes, and treatment.

Audience and Approach

While this book is directed to experienced massage therapists, the content is appropriate and useful for manual therapists of all kinds: sport chiropractors, athletic trainers, sport physicians, and other clinicians in sports medicine who work with patients recovering from soft tissue injuries. From the outset, we are assuming that the reader will be familiar with the principles of assessment, will be experienced at palpation, and will have a working knowledge of musculoskeletal anatomy (origins, insertions, and actions).

Organization

The book is divided into three parts. Part I reviews foundational knowledge that every practitioner should be familiar with. Chapter 1 defines sports massage and discusses clinical reasoning and why using clinical reasoning is critical to the evaluation and treatment of musculoskeletal injuries. Chapter 1 also includes a review and discussion of current concepts in evidence-based practice and pain science and their impact on the sports massage therapist. Chapter 2 provides a brief review of the various types and functions of soft tissues. Chapter 3 is devoted to the principles and practice of evaluation and assessment. Assessment skills are critical to designing effective treatment processes.

Part II focuses on the injury mechanisms and repair processes of soft tissues followed by a discussion of manual treatment techniques. Chapter 4 discusses the injury and repair process of soft tissues, including nerves. Chapter 4 also includes a discussion of the pros and cons of using cryotherapy as part of the treatment for both acute and chronic injuries. Chapter 5 is devoted to a detailed discussion of the various techniques used in clinical sports massage to obtain positive results in client treatment sessions.

Part III addresses, in detail, many of the most common soft tissue injuries treated by clinical sports massage therapists. Chapter 6 focuses on the lower extremity and covers ten conditions, including IT band syndrome, tendinopathies of the hamstrings, patella, and Achilles tendon, and groin strain. Chapter 7 focuses on the upper extremity and details assessment and treatment for four conditions, including rotator cuff injuries, bicipital tendinopathy, and tennis and golfer's elbow.

Chapter 8 separately addresses five common nerve entrapment syndromes, including conditions such as thoracic outlet syndrome, carpal tunnel syndrome, and piriformis syndrome.

The combination of more than 65 illustrations and 190 photographs provides practitioners with clear, precise guidance for using the assessment and treatment protocols for selected conditions.

We hope the collective knowledge and experience distilled in these pages will be a valuable resource for clinical practitioners everywhere. And we encourage practitioners to seek live, in-person learning environments in which to hone their practical skills.

INFORMED CONSENT

Based on the accumulation of information and insight gained through practices in this book, the practitioner is prepared to discuss treatment options with the client. However, before treatment begins, the client must understand and provide informed consent. Informed consent means that the practitioner has explained the massage techniques to be used, how long the treatment program is expected to take, what if any home program will be involved, and how the treatment may affect the client's activity level.

ACKNOWLEDGMENTS

Writing a book cannot occur in a vacuum, unlike the popular image of writers toiling away in lonely seclusion. It truly takes "all-hands-on-deck" to produce a print book like the one you're holding.

First and foremost, a million thanks to my wife of over 30 years, Treeanna MacHardy, for her love, support, and understanding as I focused my attention on the research and writing for this book that took many hours away from time we could have been spending together, not to mention the many chores and household tasks that languished on the to-do list, waiting for me to get to them when I had a free minute.

My collaborators at Human Kinetics have been tremendous, including my editorial team: acquisitions editor, Michelle Maloney, developmental editor, Laura Pulliam, and managing editor, Dominique Moore. Special thanks to Keri Evans who designed the book cover, to Denise Lowry, who graciously worked through a number of designs with me and Michelle until we found the right combination of color, line, and graphics, and to Heidi Richter for her excellent illustrations found throughout the book.

Special thanks to the HK photo department, including Doug Fink and Amy Rose, who organized and supervised the photo shoot and with whom it has been my pleasure to work for many years. Jason Allen is the patient and thorough HK photographer who skillfully captured the photos that demonstrate the work we're presenting here. Greg Henness handled the camera and sound for the video interviews Doug and I recorded to help promote the book.

Thanks also to Taylia Tyo, Keybeck Song, Stacie Bowden, and Scott Barber, the models who cheerfully and patiently followed myriad directions for position changes, as well as hopping on and off the treatment table numerous times so we could move it to the best light for the photo.

I have been blessed to know and work with many dedicated sports massage therapists over the last 38 years. Some of these colleagues have been gracious enough to fulfill my request for case studies to use as illustrative examples of sports massage in the care of athletic injuries. I owe tremendous thanks for their contributions to Delaney Farmer, George Glass, Mike Grafstein, Gay Koopman, Charles McGrosky, Michael Moore, Kirk Nelson, Mary Riley, Esteban Ruvalcaba, Bori Suryani, Molly Verschingel, and Earl Wenk.

Part I

Foundational Knowledge

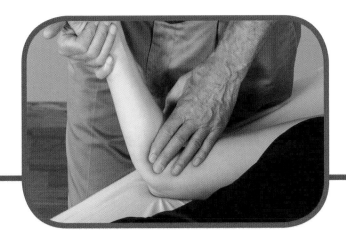

Chapter 1

Concepts and Principles

Sports massage as a distinct style of practice continues to be one of the fastest growing segments of the massage therapy profession. Sports massage can be defined as the skilled application of specific massage techniques, including range-of-motion (ROM) movements or stretching, to achieve specific goals when treating clients who participate in regular physical activity. Sports massage is usually divided into three categories:

1. Massage for injury care
2. Event massage (before, during, and after)
3. Training and maintenance massage

Massage for injury care is rehabilitative and clinically focused. Event massage does not typically include rehabilitative work, but it is used to help an athlete prepare just prior to competition (pre-event massage), to maintain readiness during a multi-event competition (inter-event massage), and to recover following competition (post-event massage). Training/maintenance massage is employed to assist the athlete during their normal training cycle to enhance recovery and to address ROM issues and muscle imbalances that may contribute to the development of overuse injuries. Specific goals and hands-on techniques are associated with each of these categories; some are the same across all categories, and some are applied in only one category. Overall sports massage goals include improving neuromuscular balance and flexibility, reducing muscle soreness and pain, and rehabilitating soft tissue injuries. Many resources exist for learning more about sports massage for event work and for training and maintenance massage. This book focuses on massage for injury care: the evaluation and treatment of neuromuscular injuries. To achieve this aim, the sports massage therapist must bring together a knowledge of injury pathology, a deep grasp of anatomy and physiology, skilled assessment using client history, ROM and manual muscle testing, orthopedic tests, and careful palpation, all filtered through a process of clinical reasoning to determine the best approach to treatment.

The Process of Clinical Reasoning

Clinical reasoning is the ability to compile and organize information gained from taking a client history and performing a thorough examination in order to develop an effective massage treatment plan. According to Fritz (2013, p. 131), "Therapeutic massage practitioners must be able to gather information effectively, analyze that information to make decisions about the type and appropriateness of an intervention, and evaluate and justify the benefits derived from the intervention."

Clinical reasoning is both an art and a science, developed through continual practice and study. The art of clinical reasoning requires a combination of deductive reasoning based on information gathering and practical experience that allows the practitioner to recognize symptom patterns during the client examination. The science of clinical reasoning includes the integration of the best available evidence (both research and experiential) when making treatment decisions, including the decision about whether to treat the client or refer them to another professional.

Treatment Decisions

Knowing when not to treat is an important component of the clinical reasoning process for sports massage therapists and all clinically oriented practitioners and is a skill deepened with clinical experience. According to Jurch (2015, p. 9),

> One major benefit of having a systematic way to gather information is to determine whether massage therapy will truly benefit the athlete. The process of treating specific musculoskeletal disorders begins first with knowing what not to treat. As healthcare practitioners, therapists have a duty to provide proper care, even if that means referring athletes to other healthcare providers. We must be able to recognize situations that are outside our scope of practice; when to modify treatments; or when the use of modalities other than massage may be more beneficial. In order to accomplish this, there must be a foundation of knowledge from which to build.

Lens of Bias

The clinically oriented sports massage practitioner must be aware of the "lens of bias" effect (also known as the confirmation bias) when it comes to injury care and management. Massage therapists, and indeed all health care providers, tend to view a condition through the lens of their discipline. Because massage therapists deal primarily with the soft tissues, the tendency is to view all conditions as soft tissue based and to assess and treat them accordingly. The error in this approach stems from ignoring or devaluing client history or symptoms that do not fit the treatment model and continuing to pursue treatment strategies that seem to prove the initial assessment. For example, it's not uncommon for an athlete to self-diagnose foot pain as plantar fasciitis and to seek massage treatment for relief. Plantar fasciitis is a common soft tissue condition characterized by pain on the bottom of the foot, especially during the first few steps after waking or after sitting for a long time. The pain then tends to decrease with additional movement. A practitioner's confirmation bias would tend to ignore factors that do not fit the plantar fasciitis picture, even though plantar pain can be caused by a number of other conditions, such as Baxter's neuropathy, an entrapment condition of the inferior calcaneal nerve under the medial arch of the foot.

When treatment for plantar fasciitis does not yield results, the practitioner who has succumbed to bias will fail to look at other potential causes of the client's ongoing pain. An experienced practitioner will apply clinical reasoning skills to account for all of the client's history and symptoms, paying special attention to those symptoms that do not fit the plantar fasciitis hypothesis, such as weakness of the abductor digiti minimi or pain with palpation of the abductor digiti minimi or along the medial arch of the foot where the nerve is likely to be compressed (figure 1.1). These details are critical because common massage therapy treatments for plantar fasciitis may aggravate Baxter's neuropathy (figure 1.2).

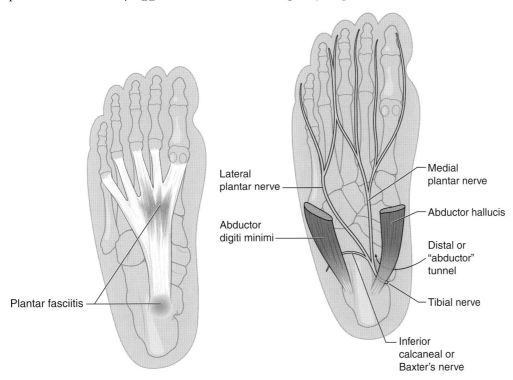

FIGURE 1.1 Typical plantar fasciitis pain sites.

FIGURE 1.2 Baxter's neuropathy pain locations.

Clinical reasoning doesn't stop after the initial client intake. As Jurch (2015, p. 9) has written,

> Formulating a treatment plan is an ongoing process for each athlete. It involves a constant sequence of assessing, treating, reassessing, and either continuing with the same treatments or trying something different. This requires therapists to continually use all of their resources to provide the most effective therapy possible.

Evidence-Based Practice (EBP)

Increasingly, massage therapists who treat injuries are utilizing an evidence-based, or evidence-informed, approach to treatment. Clinical reasoning is one element of evidence-based treatment. According to Duke University (2014, p. 2),

EBP is the integration of clinical expertise, patient values, and the best research evidence into the decision-making process for patient care. Clinical expertise refers to the clinician's cumulated experience, education and clinical skills. The patient brings to the encounter his or her own personal preferences and unique concerns, expectations, and values. The best research evidence is usually found in clinically relevant research that has been conducted using sound methodology.

Although this definition is directed at medical professionals, other health care providers—including massage therapists—have adopted or adapted the model to their own professions. One of the hallmarks of EBP is the emphasis on research evidence to support clinical decision making, especially evidence from randomized-control trials (RCTs) and systematic reviews (SRs). Many practitioners have expressed concern that this narrow focus on RCTs and SRs ignores other, equally applicable, forms of evidence. As a result, many practitioners embrace the concept of evidence-informed practice.

Soo Liang Ooi and colleagues, of the Centre for Complementary and Alternative Medicine in Singapore, coauthored a research study (2018, p. 326) that examined the attitudes of Australian practitioners toward evidence-informed practice. According to their findings,

> Critics of evidence-based practice have argued that information used to make clinical decisions should not be restricted to evidence collected from intervention research but should be inclusive of a wider range of research methods, such as cohort studies, qualitative studies, as well as clinical case reports, so that practitioners can use them in creative ways throughout the intervention process. Practices are not "based" exclusively on evidence but rather the practitioners become knowledgeable and "informed" by evidence.

The challenge for practitioners, of course, is to be able to keep up with the plethora of research, case studies, and reviews that appear in the literature while still being able to manage a massage therapy practice. Dr. Paul M. Finch, director of education for the Sutherland-Chan School of Massage Therapy in Toronto, Canada, and education editor for the *International Journal of Therapeutic Massage and Bodywork*, authored a paper in which he advocates for the "evidence funnel" approach to help sort out and narrow the amount of reading necessary for a practitioner to stay current with the most relevant information (2007). Several online resources are available to help massage therapists stay up to date on massage-related research articles, research reviews, and abstracts without the need for subscriptions to individual journals. A list of online research resources is included at the back of the book.

Pain Science

An explosion of research on pain in recent years has led to new insights into, as well as great confusion about, the origins of pain, the connections between injury and pain, and the psychological and social contributions to the perception of pain. This broadened knowledge of the complexity of pain has also affected the way manual therapy practitioners approach their work with clients.

By contrast, as the understanding of the mechanisms of pain perception and pain generation has progressed, many researchers and practitioners have reframed the discussion of pain in relation to injury by emphasizing that pain is a complex experience, involving many parts of the brain, and that pain perception is influenced by psychosocial factors that include previous pain experiences, thoughts and feelings about previous pain experiences, emotional states, and even personal relationships. These elements of the pain experience have been recognized for years but have been downplayed in favor of a pathomechanical model of pain that described the stimulation of pain receptors in the tissue when an injury or insult occurred there. These receptors would then stimulate the pain region of the brain, and pain would be felt. It now appears that pain receptors do not exist, but nociceptive receptors do and are stimulated by a variety of noxious stimuli, including pressure, temperature, and inflammatory markers. These receptors send signals to the brain via the spinal cord, and the brain evaluates the signal and determines whether the input is pain or not, and then outputs either the sensation of pain or something else, such as an increase in pressure or a feeling of additional warmth. What this means in practical terms for practitioners is that pain intensity does not necessarily correlate with tissue damage. Minor injuries can feel extremely painful, and severe injuries may occur with very little pain. This response is modulated by the brain and is dependent on all the biopsychosocial factors influencing the brain's final output.

In chronic pain conditions, a neural pathway can become sensitized by repeated nociceptive stimulation so that even minor noxious input can trigger output from the brain that causes the patient to feel pain. On the other hand, this does not mean that pain intensity never correlates directly with the amount of tissue damage, and it's critical for practitioners and patients to stay mindful of this fact.

Growing evidence indicates that incorporating pain neuroscience education (PNE) with manual treatment is efficacious for reducing chronic pain. The intent of PNE is to help shift the client's focus away from "my tissues are painful, so they must be injured" to realizing that the brain's perception and interpretation of stimuli emanating from the tissues may not always accurately reflect the degree of tissue damage. Encouraging a client to shift their focus away from the idea that their pain is caused by specific tissue damage has been shown to reduce chronic pain and, more importantly, to reduce pain catastrophization (magnifying the pain and feeling helpless in the presence of pain).

As practitioners and patients read and hear more about the new pain science, they may make the incorrect assumption that the oversimplified phrase "pain is in the brain" means that pain is all in your head. It's incumbent on the professionals to reassure patients that they're not making it all up (as has been the unfortunate experience of many patients). As Whitney Lowe, massage educator and author, has written,

> I think one of the biggest obstacles and challenges for those who are carrying the torch of the emerging pain science specialty is to understand how to introduce these ideas to those for whom this view is new. Too often I have seen and heard pain science enthusiasts speak to others with condescension and arrogance. As a teacher I clearly recognize how that produces an immediate degree of defensiveness in a student and that is a significant obstacle to learning. (Lowe 2017, p. 1)

Because knowledge about pain perception continues to emerge and evolve, the other clear message for practitioners and patients is that our prior knowledge and experience about pain and treating patients in pain is not suddenly obsolete or ineffective. "It isn't necessary to throw out all of the valuable learning and clinical experience we have already built upon. But maybe we look at these things through a different set of glasses" (Lowe 2017, p. 1). It is incumbent on sports massage practitioners to discuss with clients the current research about pain and how those research findings will affect the treatment strategies proposed in their particular case.

Summary

This opening chapter has been an overview of the concepts and principles employed in the evaluation and treatment of common soft tissue injuries by sports massage practitioners and manual therapists. Injury care and management is one category of the sports massage specialty and requires a deep commitment to gaining a broad-based knowledge of injury mechanisms, the anatomy and physiology involved, and the ability to carefully evaluate the injured client. This foundational knowledge is combined with information acquired from the client history and examination and used in a process of clinical reasoning to aid the practitioner in developing an appropriate treatment plan or in deciding to refer the client to another professional for further evaluation or treatment.

Throughout this evaluation process, the sports massage therapist must be cognizant of an inherent bias toward assuming that soft tissues are the cause of the client's signs and symptoms and is encouraged to incorporate EBP principles when making treatment decisions. An understanding of emerging knowledge in pain science is a critical component of EBP. The practitioner with a solid grasp of the complexity of the pain experience is able to convey this knowledge to injured clients in a way that helps them understand that their pain intensity is not always related to the severity of their injury and that their pain experience is real and not all in their head. The client also needs to know that the sports massage interventions may have not only a mechanical effect on the soft tissues treated but also a profound effect on the overall nervous system in the control and resolution of their pain.

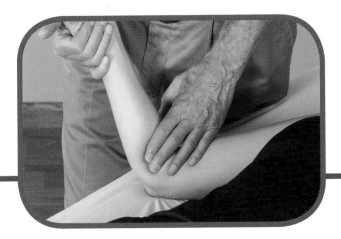

Chapter 2

Reviewing Soft Tissue Types

In recent years, a significant amount of research has focused on the various soft tissue structures of the human body. These findings have broadened and deepened our understanding of both the structure and function of these tissues. This research has also caused a shift in the way we think about the neuromuscular system, how the various neural and soft tissues interact with one another, and what happens when we perform massage therapy techniques. In the descriptions throughout the chapter, we start with the classic definitions of each tissue type and then expand to include a broad overview of new information that affects our overall understanding of their role.

Connective Tissue

Collagen is the most abundant protein in the body and is the primary structural component of connective tissue, which is considered to be the building block of all the soft tissues. Connective tissue is composed of both collagen and elastic fibers embedded in a jellylike extracellular matrix that acts as a lubricant for the fibers.

Connective tissue can be categorized as loose or dense and as regular or irregular, depending on its composition (see figure 2.1). It exhibits excellent tensile strength and is relatively inextensible. The elastic fibers in connective tissue coil and recoil like a spring and help return stretched tissue back to its original shape. The ratio of collagen and elastic fibers in different tissues varies depending on whether they need more strength or more elasticity.

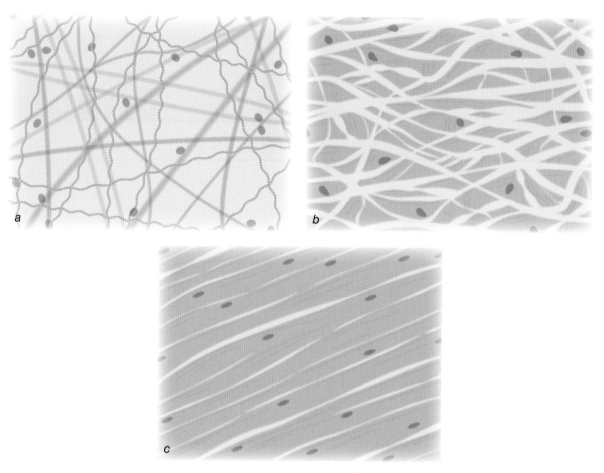

FIGURE 2.1   Connective tissue can be *(a)* loose, *(b)* dense and irregular, or *(c)* dense and regular, depending on its specific composition as well as its location and function.
© Human Kinetics

Fascia

In traditional anatomy texts, fascia has been regarded as no more than a wrapper that serves to protect and separate the "important" structures, such as muscles, tendons, ligaments, and organs. Our understanding of the role and importance of fascia has dramatically expanded as a result of intense research in this area.

Fascia is made up of various types of connective tissue and surrounds and connects every muscle and organ, forming a continuity throughout the body (see figure 2.2). Fascia varies in shape, density, and thickness according to its location in the body and the functional stresses placed on it. Although traditional anatomists believed that fascia was merely a passive form of connective tissue, research has revealed that fascia has the ability to contract and relax, contains sensory organs such as proprioceptors and mechanoreceptors, and is well innervated (Willard, Vleeming, and Schuenke 2012).

When we perform an activity, we affect and are affected by the fascial tissues and can only separate them from muscles, tendons, and ligaments as a way to learn about them. Dutch physician and anatomist Jaap van der Wal has written extensively on the need to approach the structure and function of fascia from an architectural, or functional, viewpoint rather than the classic anatomical, or dissection, model. He makes the case that the traditional study of anatomy, dividing the musculoskeletal system into separate structures such as bones, joints, muscles, and ligaments denies

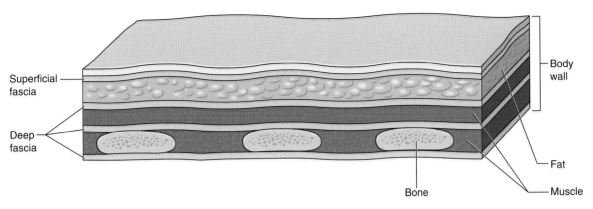

FIGURE 2.2 Superficial fascia lies just below the skin. Deep (or investing) fascia surrounds individual muscles; divides groups of muscles; and surrounds bones, organs, and nerves throughout the body.

the connectivity and continuity of these elements. He states that, "architectural and mechanical spatial relationships between the various tissue components of the musculoskeletal system reveal functional units that go across the traditional anatomic entities of bones, joints, and muscles" (van der Wal 2009, p.10).

Remember this broader view of the functional relationships of the entire musculoskeletal system during the upcoming discussion, which is based on the traditional anatomical model of discrete components such as ligaments, tendons, muscles, and nerves. The words of the late Dr. Leon Chaitow are worth noting here:

> One of the surprising features resulting from current fascia research (and there is an awful lot of it) is how little our increased understanding of fascia's functions has changed what manual therapists actually do—or need to do. Rather, I believe, greater fascial awareness and understanding helps most therapists to do what they already do, more effectively, rather than having to relearn their skills. (Chaitow 2015, p.1)

For example, this greater awareness of fascial continuity impacts the treatment of injury to fascial structures, such as the IT band, as described in chapter 6. Additionally, the sports massage therapist who maintains a global view of the fascial continuities incorporates treatments that address the structures surrounding the area of the injury, even while more specific hands-on work focuses on specific areas to achieve results.

Ligaments

Traditional anatomy texts describe ligaments as fibrous bands made up of regular dense connective tissue that attach bones to each other. In simple terms, they hold joints together. Ligaments are composed primarily of collagen bundles in parallel, with a mixture of elastic fibers and fine collagen fibers interwoven. This arrangement creates tissue that is pliable enough to allow freedom of motion at the joint and strong enough to resist stretching forces. They provide the majority of resistance at the end range of a joint's movement. If they are repeatedly overstretched, they lose their ability to return to their normal length, compromising joint stability. This creates joint laxity and sets the stage for joint sprain, or even rupture of the ligament.

Traditionally, ligaments are considered to be passive structures, merely resisting mechanical forces on the joint, and only in the positions that specifically load the ligamentous fibers (see figure 2.3). In keeping with the concept that all connective tissue structures are intimately connected, van der Wal (2009) describes extensive anatomical study that reveals that ligaments are in fact continuous with the fascial sleeves in which the muscles that cross a joint also run. He describes them as being in series with the muscle tissue and not as parallel but separate entities. He declares that ligaments actively provide support to the joint structure throughout the joint's range of motion as part of a connective tissue stability system. Van der Wal coined the term *dynament* (dynamic ligament) to more clearly refer to the function of ligaments that cross synovial joints (see figure 2.4). This updated view

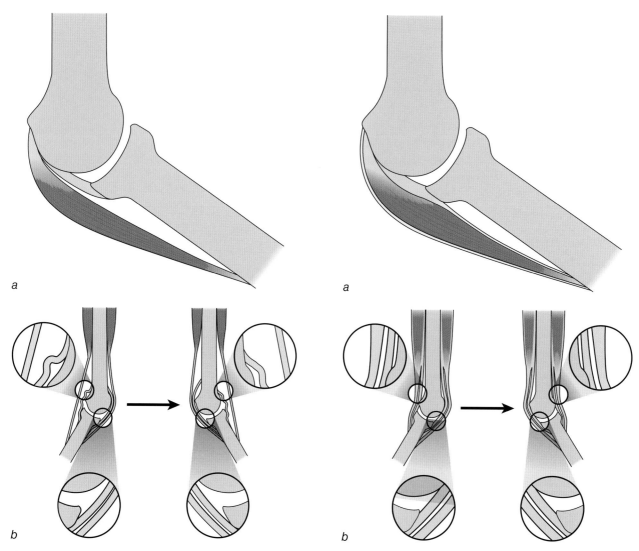

FIGURE 2.3 Ligaments are traditionally described as *(a)* running in parallel to the muscles and *(b)* functioning primarily when under tension at the end of a joint's ROM.

Adapted by permission from J. Van der Wal, "The Architecture of the Connective Tissue in the Musculoskeletal System: An Often Overlooked Functional Parameter as to Proprioception in the Locomotor Apparatus," *International Journal of Therapeutic Massage & Bodywork* 2, no. 4 (2009): 9–23.

FIGURE 2.4 *(a)* van der Wal coined the term *dynament* (dynamic ligament) to describe muscles and ligaments that run in series with each other. *(b)* The dynament is under tension and provides support in all joint positions.

Adapted by permission from J. Van der Wal, "The Architecture of the Connective Tissue in the Musculoskeletal System: An Often Overlooked Functional Parameter as to Proprioception in the Locomotor Apparatus," *International Journal of Therapeutic Massage & Bodywork* 2, no. 4 (2009): 9–23.

of ligaments as intimately connected and active with the muscle–tendon units that cross the same joint influences the treatment of ligament injuries such as lateral ankle sprains, described in chapter 6.

Tendons

In light of the discussion of fascia in the previous paragraphs, it must be acknowledged that this discussion of tendons as separate structures is merely an artificial construct to help study and discuss them. In traditional anatomy terms, tendons connect muscles to bones. Tendons are made up of closely packed bundles of collagen fibers that run in parallel along the line of pull exerted by the muscle (see figure 2.5). The primary function of tendons is to transmit the contraction forces of muscles to bones, thereby creating movement. It's also clear from fascia research that muscle–tendon units do not act individually, but that contraction forces of muscles are spread through the fascial network to adjacent structures (Maas and Sandercock 2010). This fascial research reinforces the importance of including treatment for the tissues surrounding an identified injury.

Although tendons can sustain acute injuries such as rupture or laceration (as can occur when a sharp knife slips while chopping vegetables and cuts a finger to the bone), the most common tendon injuries are those resulting from overuse. These overuse injuries to tendons used to be categorized as inflammatory conditions and called tendinitis (or tendonitis). Because a body of research over the past 30 years has indicated that many of these chronic tendon injuries are the result of tissue degradation and disorganization, with little or no inflammation present, these are now referred to as tendinosis or tendinopathy (Li and Hua 2016; Rudavsky and Cook 2014).

Interestingly, the pendulum has begun to swing back toward viewing inflammation as a component, although not the primary cause, in the development of

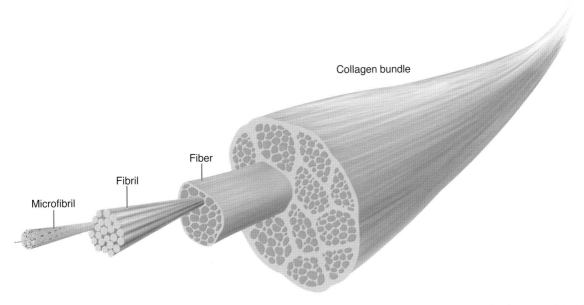

FIGURE 2.5 Tendons consist of bundles of collagen fibers that converge from the layers of fascia that surround their muscles.

chronic tendinopathy. Rees and colleagues (2014) argue that researchers and practitioners would do well to place more emphasis on incorporating anti-inflammatory strategies when treating chronic tendinopathy. Read more about tendon injuries in chapters 6 and 7 where the treatment for several common tendinopathy conditions are discussed.

Muscles

Muscle tissue is composed of closely packed contractile proteins called myofibrils that have the ability to shorten, causing the muscle to contract. This contraction force is transmitted to the muscle tendons (and surrounding fascial sheets), which pull on the bones, causing movement.

Muscles are classified into three main types: smooth, cardiac, and skeletal. Our main interest in this discussion is skeletal muscle. Skeletal muscles connect to bones via tendons (and fascia) and act as movers or as stabilizers (see figure 2.6). Skeletal muscles are sometimes referred to as voluntary muscles because they're under conscious control. Skeletal muscle tissue is made up of individual muscle fibers, each wrapped in a connective tissue layer called the endomysium. Groups of these individual fibers, called fascicles, are bundled and held together by a second layer of connective tissue called the perimysium. Finally, bundles of fascicles are grouped and held together by a third layer of connective tissue called the epimysium (part of the overall deep fascia network). This epimysium layer surrounding the entire muscle converges at each end of the muscle belly to form the tendons that attach the muscle to the bones via the periosteum.

Skeletal muscles can be injured in a variety of ways, including acute trauma such as rupture or laceration, or more chronically as a result of overuse or overload. Skeletal muscle has the ability to regenerate after minor injuries, but even simple strains can heal poorly, leaving the tissues vulnerable to reinjury. According to Garg and colleagues (2015, p. 2),

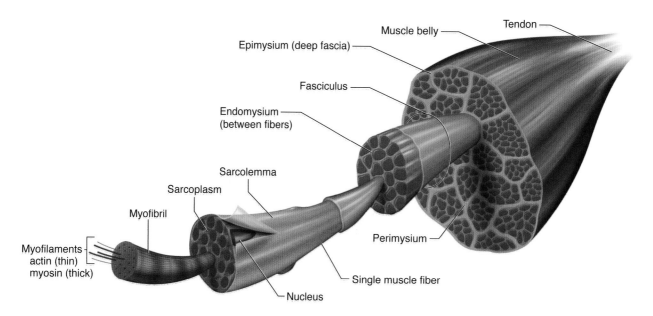

FIGURE 2.6   Skeletal muscle is made up of bundles inside bundles.

The major impediment to optimal muscle healing after any injury is fibrosis, defined as an abnormal and unresolvable, chronic overproliferation of extracellular matrix (ECM) components. Fibrosis interferes with muscle regeneration, causes a loss in muscle function and alters the tissue environment causing increased susceptibility to reinjury.

Sports massage techniques can be used to help minimize the development of dysfunctional fibrosis in injured skeletal muscle. In their paper in the *Journal of Athletic Training* (2014, p. 266), Christine Waters-Banker, PhD and ATC, and colleagues stated that,

> Massage has the potential to attenuate the inflammatory process, facilitate early recovery, and provide pain relief from muscular injuries. In this hypothesis-driven paper, we integrate the concept of mechanotransduction with the application of massage to explore beneficial mechanisms. By altering signaling pathways involved with the inflammatory process, massage may decrease secondary injury, nerve sensitization, and collateral sprouting, resulting in increased recovery from damage and reduction or prevention of pain.

Nerves

For purposes of discussion and study, the nervous system is usually divided into the central nervous system, which includes nerves of the brain and spinal cord, and the peripheral nervous system (PNS), which includes nerves outside of the central nervous system.

A typical peripheral nerve is made up of groups of nerve fibers (see figure 2.7). At the deepest level, each nerve fiber (the axon), is actually a bundle of neurofibrils, surrounded by a layer of loose connective tissue called the endoneurium. These axons are grouped into fascicles and wrapped in a layer of connective tissue called the perineurium. At the most superficial level, the fascicles are wrapped in a layer of dense connective tissue called the epineurium, containing the blood vessels and lymphatics that nourish the nerve.

Peripheral nerves are divided into three categories based on the direction their impulses travel:

1. *Afferent (sensory) nerves* carry signals via sensory neurons to the central nervous system, for example, from mechanoreceptors in the skin or from other proprioceptors in the muscle bellies, tendons, and so on.

2. *Efferent (motor) nerves* communicate from the central nervous system via motor neurons to their target muscles and glands.

3. *Mixed nerves* contain both afferent and efferent axons, so they conduct both incoming sensory information and outgoing motor impulses in the same bundle.

Nerves are susceptible to injury as a result of too much pressure (crushing, compression and entrapment, repetitive stress), they can suffer lacerations or

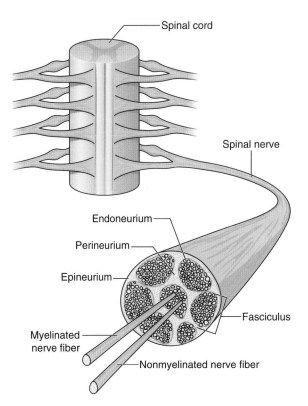

FIGURE 2.7 Similar to skeletal muscle, each nerve axon is wrapped in connective tissue (endoneurium), groups of axons are bundled by connective tissue into fascicles (perineurium), and groups of fascicles are bundled by connective tissue (epineurium) to form the nerve fiber.

tears, and they can be subject to overstretching. In many cases, sports massage can be a useful adjunct to overall treatment for chronic nerve entrapment conditions such as carpal tunnel syndrome and thoracic outlet syndrome. Nerve injury and treatment is discussed more fully in chapter 8.

Summary

This chapter has reviewed and defined the major types of soft tissue in the body. This brief overview of the structure and function of collagen, fascia, ligaments, tendons, muscles, and nerves is meant as a refresher for the experienced sports massage practitioner. For a more in-depth study of these tissues, consider exploring *Structure and Function of the Musculoskeletal System, Second Edition*, by James Watkins, and *Skeletal Muscle: Form and Function, Second Edition*, by Brian MacIntosh, Phillip Gardiner, and Alan McComas.

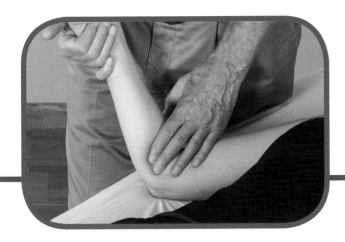

Chapter 3

Principles of Assessment

Accurate assessment is vital for properly treating soft tissue injuries. The goal of the assessment process is to locate the structure or structures responsible for the client's pain. Although massage therapists are not legally qualified to diagnose a condition or injury, the profession's scope of practice includes the right to assess a client to determine whether massage therapy is appropriate treatment for her condition or whether the client needs to be referred to another practitioner. This chapter is intended as a detailed refresher for the experienced sports massage therapist. It may also serve as a thorough introduction to the principles of assessment for the therapist who may not have studied the topic during their initial training as a sports massage therapist.

HOPS Method

Thorough evaluation includes several steps that can be summarized by the acronym HOPS: history, observation, palpation, and special tests. Table 3.1 contains examples of the types of information collected in each category, but it is by no

TABLE 3.1 HOPS Evaluation Summary

Take a thorough history (subjective findings)	Clinical observation of what can be seen, heard, or felt (objective findings)	Palpation (to support objective findings)	Special tests
• Consider the most likely injury. • Ask the right questions. • Consider referred pain.	• Swelling or atrophy • Abnormal color (bruising, redness, paleness) • Postural issues • Altered gait mechanics • Facial expressions	• Heat or cold • Crepitus or grinding • Point tenderness • Muscle spasm	• Joint range of motion • Muscle strength and function • Active, passive, and resisted movements

means a comprehensive list. The HOPS process provides the practitioner with a systematic, repeatable method for evaluating injuries.

History

An accurate history of the problem presented by the athlete is essential for determining a proper course of treatment. Some conditions have a characteristic pattern of onset and symptoms that can be ascertained from the history. For instance, if an athlete reporting a knee injury describes hearing a pop in his knee at the time of injury, accompanied by the knee giving way, this combination is characteristic of a meniscal or ligament injury, or both.

Taking a thorough history is the beginning of the deductive process that eventually leads to a working hypothesis of what the injury may be and whether it's a condition that would benefit from sports massage therapy. The information acquired in the history helps direct the next steps in the HOPS evaluation.

The history should include, but is not limited to, these questions:

Gathering background information on the injury or complaint

- What happened? Where? When?
- Do you have a previous history of this injury or issues with this body part?
- Did you hear anything (e.g., popping, grinding)?
- Did you feel anything (e.g., popping, burning, joint giving way, numbness)?

Gathering information about the primary complaint

- What symptoms or complaint brought you in today?
- What symptoms are bothering you the most today?
- What were the symptoms at the time of injury?
- How would you describe the pain today (e.g., achy, sharp, burning, throbbing)?
- How would you rate today's pain on a scale from 0 to 10?
- What makes your symptoms worse?
- What makes your symptoms better?

Gathering information about previous diagnosis and treatment

Learning about a previous diagnosis and any previous treatment and its outcome helps a practitioner design a treatment plan with a greater chance of success.

- Has there been a previous diagnosis? If so, who made the diagnosis and what was it?
- Has there been previous treatment? If so, what was done and by whom?
- What were the results of the treatment?

Observation

Observation is generally limited to what the practitioner can see, feel, or hear, as opposed to what the client reports subjectively. When possible, quantifying the finding in some way is valuable for documenting results. For instance, a swollen ankle could be noted as mild, moderate, or severe. Even better, one could measure the ankle circumference (comparing to the uninjured side). After treatment, changes can be documented to show the effectiveness of the treatment administered. During observation, look for the following:

- Swelling or atrophy
- Abnormal color (bruising, redness, paleness)
- Postural issues such as an antalgic position, holding, guarding
- Altered gait mechanics, for example limping
- Heat or cold (note color changes in the skin due to heat or cold)
- The sound of crepitus or grinding
- Facial expressions that could indicate pain

Palpation

The palpatory examination is guided by the findings gathered from the history and observation. Palpation is performed on the uninjured side first (to obtain a benchmark for normal) and then proceeds cautiously on the injured side.

The palpation portion of the HOPS evaluation is the discrete use of the fingers, thumbs, or back of the hand to help determine the quality of the soft tissues. Palpation is performed to identify the feel and quality of the injured area, with special attention to previous observations such as swelling and temperature changes, as well as to muscle spasm, crepitus, and significant point tenderness. Palpation may also include passive ROM to get a sense of the condition of the movement quality of joint (e.g., spongy, springy, etc.). Later in the assessment process, palpation will play a key role in determining exactly where massage and additional techniques, such as stretching, will be administered.

Special Tests

In general, this portion of the assessment examines passive and active joint range of motion and muscle activation. The aim of accurate evaluation is to locate the structure responsible for the athlete's pain. This is accomplished using a variety of tests to stress the suspected tissues. Healthy tissue is expected to function without pain or weakness. When injured tissue is placed under stress, pain will increase (especially the pain that brought the athlete in for evaluation) or the tissue will be weak, or both.

Assessing Active, Passive, and Resisted Motion

Evaluation protocols that test active, passive, and resisted movements are intended to investigate the soft tissues that could be the source of the client's pain. These assessments, with the potential findings for each, are summarized in table 3.2 and then described in detail. As with all tests, assessment begins with the noninvolved side first, then moves to the injured side, at the joint closest to the client's pain symptoms. Depending on initial findings, testing may need to progress more globally to rule out injury above or below the suspected joint, especially if referred pain is suspected.

From a sports massage perspective, these assessments are concerned primarily with two types of soft tissue: contractile and noncontractile (also called inert tissues).

TABLE 3.2 Joint Motion Assessment Summary

Active motion	Passive motion	Resisted (isometric) motion
• Tests all the structures around the joint. • Serves as a "ballpark" test to determine which joint is at fault. • Performed by the client, with no assistance from the therapist. **Findings:** • Pain: Tested joint is causing pain. • Pain free: Other structures might be referring pain.	• Tests noncontractile tissues (ligaments, nerves, joint capsules, and bursae). • Performed by the therapist, with no assistance from the client. • Assesses the noncontractile tissues without engaging the contractile tissues. • Examines for pain, limitation, and end feel. **Findings:** • Pain: Injury present in tested tissues. • Pain free: Normal. • Abnormal end feel: See end-feel categories.	• Tests contractile tissues (muscles, tendons, and associated fascial bands) • Strong isometric contraction loads the muscle and tendon fibers without stressing the joint or the noncontractile tissues around the joint. • Specifically assesses the tissues at the suspected joint. • Examines for pain or weakness, or both. **Findings:** • Pain: Injury present in the tested tissue. • Painless weakness: Nerve conduction issue. • Pain free and strong: Normal.

Adapted from J.H. Cynax and P.J. Cynax, *Cynax's Illustrated Manual of Orthopaedic Medicine* (Oxford, OK: Butterworths, 1983), and other sources.

The active, passive, and resisted motion tests engage these tissues in different ways to help narrow the search for the cause of the athlete's symptoms.

Contractile tissues

Contractile tissues include muscles, tendons, and associated fascial bands. The muscle–tendon units are evaluated globally during active ROM testing and more specifically by using resisted (isometric) muscle tests. These tests load the muscle and tendon fibers, while minimizing stress on other structures. An increase in pain or weakness, or both, is considered a positive finding and indicates muscle strain or tendon issues in the tested muscle–tendon unit. Injuries in contractile tissues respond well to the massage techniques featured in this book.

Noncontractile tissues

Ligaments, nerves, joint capsules, and bursae are considered to be noncontractile tissues. These tissues are evaluated globally during active ROM testing and more specifically by using passive movements that test the integrity of the tissue without involving the contractile tissues. Positive findings in these tests indicate that one or more of these tissues is the site of the pain-causing lesion. Ligament sprains respond well to specific massage techniques, such as deep transverse friction. In nerve entrapment conditions, sports massage directed at the tissues that contribute to the entrapment is valuable. For the most part, injuries to bursae and capsules do not benefit from the direct application of sports massage.

The following assessments are typically performed to help determine which structures to investigate with a more detailed palpatory examination. All assessments are performed on the unaffected side first to document a baseline for their normal motion and to help allay any fears that testing the affected side will be painful.

Assessment Using Active Motion

Active motion tests all the structures around the joint. It's a general test to determine whether the search for the injury site is beginning in the right place. As the name implies, the client performs active motion, with no assistance from the therapist. Active motion is used to compare and document the ROM and quality of movement between the unaffected and the affected sides. Active motion on the unaffected side is expected to be within normal range for the joints being tested, and the movement quality is expected to appear smooth and easy. Active motion on the affected side is observed and documented, noting any limitations in ROM, any parts of the motion that appear difficult, or that activate compensatory movements, and where in the motion the athlete feels pain.

For example, when an athlete complains of shoulder pain, active motion can be used to evaluate the shoulder complex, especially the rotator cuff. Figures 3.1–3.4 illustrate active flexion, extension, abduction, adduction, internal and external rotation, and horizontal abduction and adduction. The practitioner directs the client to perform these movements, starting with the uninjured side to get a sense of and document the quality and range of normal movement for this client. This normal is then used as the comparison when documenting active movement on the injured side. It's important to note that restrictions in ROM on the affected side could be caused by a variety of issues, other than a painful lesion. These include, but are not limited to, hypertrophy, hypertonicity, weakness, soft tissue scarring, the client being fearful of performing the active movement, or nerve damage preventing the muscle from contracting.

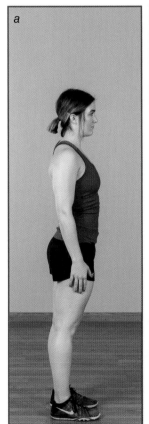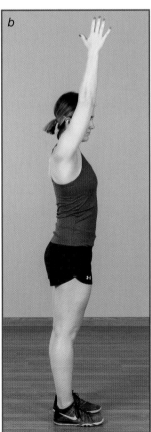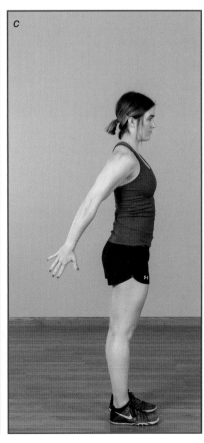

FIGURE 3.1 Normal ranges of active motion of the shoulder girdle: *(a)* neutral, *(b)* flexion, and *(c)* extension.

FIGURE 3.2 Normal ranges of active motion of the shoulder girdle: *(a)* neutral, *(b)* abduction, and *(c)* adduction.

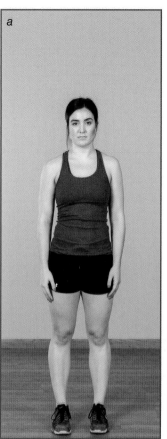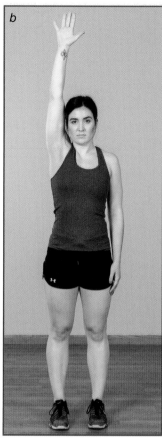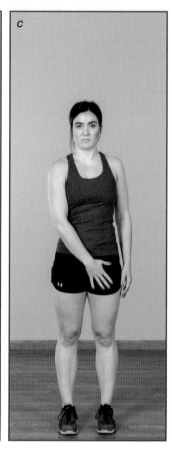

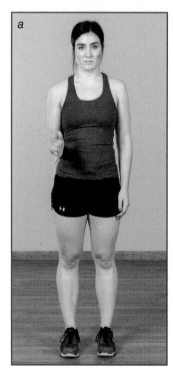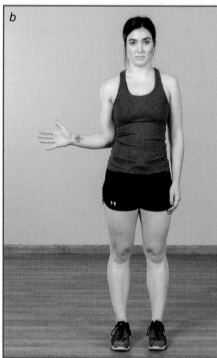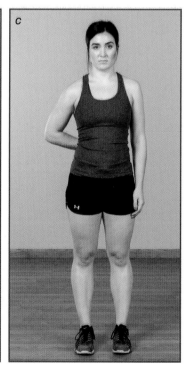

FIGURE 3.3 Normal ranges of active motion of the shoulder girdle: *(a)* neutral, *(b)* external rotation, and *(c)* internal rotation.

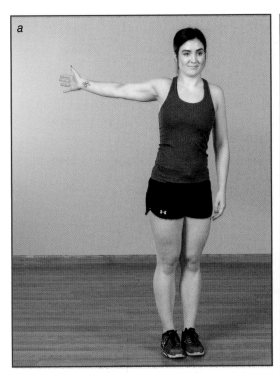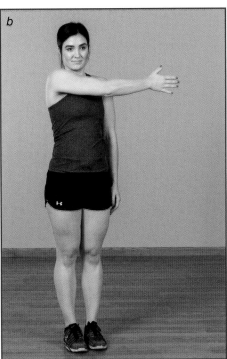

FIGURE 3.4 Normal ranges of active motion of the shoulder girdle: *(a)* horizontal abduction and *(b)* horizontal adduction.

If active testing proves to be completely pain free, this usually indicates that the source of pain is elsewhere, and the client is experiencing referred pain. Occasionally, active motion assessment will be pain free, even though further tests will elicit the pain, especially if the injury is in contractile tissue. This is because active motion often requires less force than subsequent specific tests that require the recruitment of more muscle fibers and involve the injured area enough to generate the symptoms.

Assessment Using Passive Motion

Passive motion is performed by the therapist, with no assistance from the client. Normal passive range of motion is usually greater than active range and is done bilaterally to compare the unaffected and affected sides. Continuing with the example of complaints of shoulder pain, the practitioner repeats the same set of movement tests as in the active tests, encouraging the client not to help so as to get a true reading of the quality and range of pain-free passive movement available. Passive motion on the unaffected side is expected to be within normal range for the joints being tested, and the movement quality is expected to feel smooth and easy. Passive motion on the affected side is performed and documented, noting any limitations in ROM, any parts of the motion that appear difficult, or that activate compensatory movements, and where in the motion the athlete feels pain. Figure 3.5 illustrates a few passive motion assessments.

Passive motion assesses the noncontractile tissues without engaging the contractile tissues. Increased pain during passive testing but not during resisted tests (the next step) usually indicates that noncontractile tissue is injured. However, at or near the ends of range, passive motion may cause pain by stretching injured contractile tissue or by pinching it against bone.

FIGURE 3.5 Selected passive movement assessments of the shoulder complex: *(a)* flexion, *(b)* extension, *(c)* external rotation, *(d)* internal rotation.

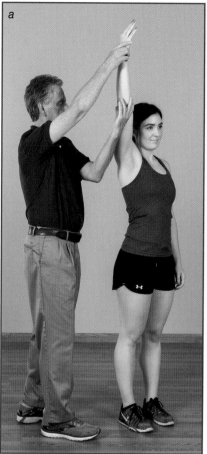
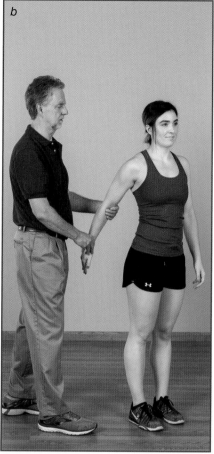
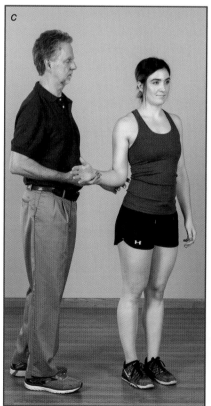
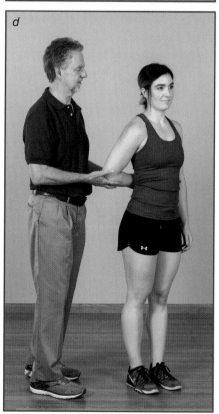

Assessment Using Manual Resistive Tests

Resisted motion is used to specifically assess contractile tissues (muscle, tendon, and associated fascial bands). This isometric assessment is conducted by asking the client to perform a strong isometric contraction that isolates and loads the muscle–tendon unit while the therapist holds the joint in neutral to avoid stressing the noncontractile tissues around the joint.

A finding of weakness or an increase in pain (as the client came in with some pain already) are positive for the tissue tested and indicate muscle strain or tendon issues, or both. To perform a manual resistive test and properly assess the contractile tissue around a joint, follow these steps:

1. Position the limb so the joint is at midrange (neutral). Manual resistive testing done at or near a joint's end of range could also stress the noncontractile tissues, providing unclear results. Proper positioning isolates the specific muscle–tendon unit to be tested.

2. Provide matching resistance as the client isometrically contracts the muscle being tested, starting gradually and building to a full contraction. Continuing with shoulder assessment; if ROM tests indicate rotator cuff injury, the manual resistive tests are used to isolate and assess each of the four rotator cuff muscles. To test the supraspinatus (the most commonly injured cuff muscle), the practitioner positions the client with the arm hanging at the side. The practitioner then stabilizes the arm at the elbow and directs the client to slowly attempt to abduct the arm while the practitioner provides matching resistance to prevent the arm from moving (see figure 3.6). One of the following results should occur:

    a. If the muscle tested is strong and pain free, there is no overt injury. Continue testing other suspected muscles. Even if no overt injury is found through testing, a subclinical condition may be discovered when performing the palpation assessment.

    b. If the pain the client is complaining of increases, stop the test. The lesion is probably contained in that muscle or tendon. Additional pain symptoms may arise during these tests. These additional symptoms may be indicative of other issues in conjunction with the primary complaint. Make a note of them and continue testing for the presenting complaint.

    c. If the muscle is weak but pain free, there may be a possible nerve conduction problem, which should be evaluated by a qualified physician.

3. If the test causes increased pain, begin the palpation assessment of the tested muscle–tendon unit for the exact site of the injury, using pain reports from the client and tissue assessment to guide the exam. Pain will be the greatest at the exact site of the lesion.

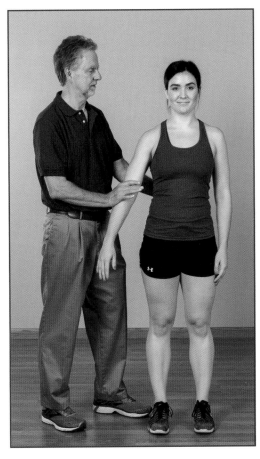

FIGURE 3.6 Manual resistive test for the supraspinatus.

It's important to note that sports injuries often involve both contractile and noncontractile tissues. If an increase in pain occurs with both passive motion tests and resisted motion tests, then it may be that both noncontractile and contractile tissue is injured. It may also mean that the noncontractile tissue is healthy, but the contractile elements are swollen and inflamed and being pinched during the passive test.

Additional Tests

Once the preliminary movement assessments have been performed, it may be useful to include additional, more specific orthopedic tests to further pinpoint the injury site. These are specialized to focus on the joint being examined and can be categorized as orthopedic or as neural tests.

Orthopedic Tests

Orthopedic assessments are used to test for specific musculoskeletal problems. A variety of orthopedic tests target specific regions of the body and many tissue types. These tests by themselves do not confirm a finding. Rather, the results must be viewed in context with the history, observation, and other assessments to get a total picture of the nature of injury. Importantly, a single positive test does not necessarily indicate a specific problem, and a single negative test does not necessarily rule out the problem. Instructions for performing specific orthopedic tests are included in the chapters that cover specific injury conditions.

Neural Tests

A variety of specialized neural tests has been developed to evaluate the peripheral nerves for mobility along their pathways, as well as possible nerve compression by soft tissue structures. Reproduction of the client's symptoms through neural testing is considered to be a positive finding for that test. Remember, a single positive test does not necessarily indicate a specific problem, and a single negative test does not necessarily rule out the problem. Instructions for performing relevant neural tests are included in the chapters that cover specific injury conditions.

Assess End Feel

Quality of motion, especially at the end of the range, is assessed through the application of mild overpressure at or near the end of passive motion. This is called *end feel*. Every joint has a normal end feel. Abnormal end feel, or normal end feel at the wrong place in the ROM, indicates injury or pathology. The ability to assess end feel improves with practice and experience.

James Cyriax, a British orthopedic physician, pioneered the discussion of end feel, and many other experts have since described different types of end feel. Cyriax wrote, "The significance of the end-feel is thus the degree to which it corresponds to or differs from what the end-feel would be if the joint were normal. Different types of end-feel imply different disorders" (Cyriax and Cyriax 1983, p.8). The following are common examples of end feel:

- *Boggy:* This is a soft and mushy feel that occurs because of joint effusion or edema. This may indicate acute swelling and inflammation. A good example would be a moderate to severe ankle inversion sprain.

- *Bony:* This is a hard stop when two bones touch each other. Elbow extension is a good example of the normal end feel being bone to bone. If the end feel of an elbow extension were not a hard stop, this would be an abnormal finding.

- *Capsular (often extended to include ligamentous):* This is typically described as a "firm but leathery" stop. Normal capsular end feel occurs when the joint capsule is the primary limiter of the end range, such as with external rotation of the shoulder.

- *Empty:* This category is used when the practitioner is unable to reach the end feel because the client stops the test due to pain or anticipated pain. In this case, there is no physical restriction to the movement, but the client is purposefully preventing movement through the full ROM. A good example of this occurs with shoulder impingement conditions, where soft tissue pain occurs before normal end feel can be achieved.

- *Muscle stretch:* The motion stops as a result of the tissue reaching the end of its stretch. This feels rubbery or slightly springy, like stretching a bicycle tire inner tube. A good example of this end feel occurs when the hip is flexed while the knee is held in extension and motion is stopped by the hamstrings. A client with extremely tight hamstrings may have a normal end feel but is well short of a normal ROM. This would indicate a condition to be treated.

- *Soft tissue approximation:* The motion stops when two masses of tissue (muscle, fat) press against each other, such as calf muscles pressing against hamstrings during knee flexion.

- *Spasm:* The movement ends abruptly, short of normal end range, and is accompanied by pain or anticipated pain. Spasm has a springy, rebound end feel that represents protective muscle guarding.

- *Springy block:* The motion stops short of normal, accompanied by a bouncy sensation, like when compressing a spring. This indicates that a loose body may be blocking the motion; it is commonly felt in the knee when a piece of floating cartilage or a torn meniscus limits knee extension.

Perpetuating Factors

Many chronic athletic injuries are characterized by elements that contribute to their inability to fully resolve. These perpetuating factors can be revealed in the client history and more thoroughly explored with conversation and observation during and after the assessment process. These factors can be broadly categorized as training factors, biomechanical factors, and equipment-related factors.

Training Factors

Elements of the athlete's training that may contribute to the presenting complaint can include activities such as the following:

- Increasing mileage or yardage (running, cycling, swimming) too rapidly
- Excessive hill running
- Improper stretching and warm-up
- Dancing en pointe

Biomechanical Factors

This category relates to the athlete's physical makeup, including compensatory patterns that may result from the following biomechanical traits:

- Overpronation
- Tight or weak hamstrings
- Pelvic imbalances
- Forward head posture
- Improper landing technique in jumping sports
- Poor swimming stroke mechanics

Equipment-Related Factors

The equipment athletes use in their sport may contribute to their condition. The practitioner needs to have a broad base of knowledge to adequately explore this category with the athlete and then know when to refer the athlete to an equipment specialist when appropriate. The following are factors to consider in this category:

- Condition of the footwear used
- Bike fit, including seat height and position of the handlebars
- Aerobic dance on unforgiving floors
- Running on concrete versus asphalt versus dirt trails

Summary

The ability to correctly assess the condition causing the symptoms an athlete is complaining of can be the difference between success or failure in the treatment of that athlete. This chapter has provided a framework for the systematic assessment of soft tissue injuries (HOPS method), as well as reminders to evaluate perpetuating factors that may prolong the recovery from injury. These assessment protocols are developed more thoroughly in the chapters that cover specific injuries commonly seen in the sports massage therapy setting.

Part II

A Closer Look at Injury and Repair

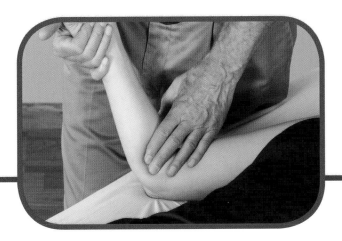

Chapter 4

Soft Tissue Injury and Repair

Sports massage therapists are primarily concerned with injury prevention through the use of maintenance massage, that is, massage performed with the aim of helping an athlete during the regular training cycle to enhance recovery, and to address physical issues that may contribute to the development of overuse injuries. However, sports massage practitioners are regularly called on by clients to evaluate and treat soft tissue injuries or complaints of pain. Although sports therapists are not legally authorized to offer a medical diagnosis, it is within their scope of practice to evaluate injuries and treat the complaints that are within their treatment capabilities.

This chapter reviews acute and chronic soft tissue injuries, discusses the classifications used to grade them, and summarizes the three stages of healing following a soft tissue injury. Additionally, an overview is provided of the current thinking concerning the use of RICE (rest, ice, compression, elevation) for acute injury management, a discussion of the causes of chronic injury, and a review of the underlying causes of nerve entrapment injuries. An understanding of these topics provides the foundational knowledge needed to implement the sports massage techniques discussed in ensuing chapters.

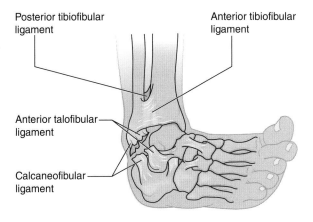

FIGURE 4.1 Lateral ankle sprain.

Acute Injuries

Acute injuries are those that occur suddenly and overload the tissue all at once. The most common acute sports injury is a lateral ankle sprain (see figure 4.1). Other examples of acute injury include muscles strains, broken bones, and joint dislocations.

Types of Acute Injuries

All acute soft tissue injuries, whether from a direct blow, an overstretch, or a tear, result in similar pathological tissue changes. Acute injury can be classified and discussed as either primary or secondary.

Primary Injury

Primary injury is the precipitating event (macrotrauma) that causes the tissue damage, tissue death, and blood seepage outside of vessels and capillaries, creating a hematoma (a mass of tissue debris and blood). The immediate application of RICE to a primary injury has been the standard protocol for many years because it has been hypothesized that the RICE strategy can greatly reduce the extent of secondary injury. This protocol has been challenged by numerous authors and practitioners recently, and the ensuing controversy is addressed in more detail later in this chapter.

Secondary Injury

Secondary injury occurs through an enlargement of the original hematoma by the addition of necrotic tissue, damaged not by the primary trauma but, secondarily, from ischemia due to reduced blood flow, reduced oxygen, and inadequate removal of metabolic waste as a result of swelling during the inflammation phase of an acute injury. Immediate application of RICE to an acute injury is still used by the majority of professionals to control inflammation and swelling. Ice has been thought to lower the metabolic needs of the healthy tissue in the vicinity of the injury site and thereby reduce the secondary tissue damage and death. Traditional thinking is that if inflammation and swelling are not controlled, the secondary injury can become worse than the original injury.

Factors Contributing to Acute Injury

Although acute injuries usually occur without warning, they are frequently the result of predisposing factors such as muscle fatigue, muscle imbalance, or other training elements that could be modified to prevent the conditions that lead to acute injury. For instance, strained muscles frequently occur because of muscle fatigue. An example is when fatigued hamstrings release more slowly following contraction. When the quadriceps contract strongly during the swing and stance phases of gait, they can actually overpower the fatigued hamstrings and cause a strain injury. Modification of an exercise program to help achieve adequate endurance and the proper strength ratio between the hamstrings and quadriceps would be a preventive measure the athlete could undertake to reduce the possibility of an acute strain to the hamstrings.

Four main factors may contribute to acute injury occurrence. It's important for the sports massage therapist to take these into account when discussing an ongoing training cycle with an athlete. Paying attention to these four controllable factors helps minimize the chances of an acute injury occurring.

1. *Excessive duration or intensity of exercise, or both.* This overwhelms the capability of the muscles, tendons, and ligaments to adapt to the stress of exercise.

2. *Inadequate strength of muscles, tendons, and ligaments.* Muscle strength increases rapidly. Tendons and ligaments build more slowly because of their limited blood supply and so are more vulnerable to injury in the early stages of an exercise program.

SPRAIN VERSUS STRAIN

Sprains and strains are acute injuries; that is, they occur suddenly as a result of an accident, a fall, or overexertion. The terms, although commonly confused, are not interchangeable.

A *sprain* is an injury to a ligament (attaches bone to bone). Because ligaments usually support a joint, a sprain will generally involve other joint structures as well as the ligament. Sprains are often accompanied by strains to one or more of the muscle–tendon units that cross the joint. A *strain* is an injury to a muscle or a tendon (attaches muscle to bone). An athlete reporting a pulled muscle is talking about a strain.

Sprains and strains are classified according to their degree of severity, as follows:

First-Degree (Grade 1) Sprain or Strain

Fibers are stretched and minimal fibers are torn. The joint is stable, with no loss of function. There may be mild to moderate pain and some swelling.

Second-Degree (Grade 2) Sprain or Strain

This category generally means that 50% of the fibers are torn. Some texts classify second degree to mean **any** tearing of fibers, from 1% to 99%. A second-degree sprain causes some joint instability and loss of full function. Muscle splinting is often present, with moderate to severe pain and swelling.

Third-Degree (Grade 3) Sprain or Strain

In a third-degree sprain or strain injury, all the fibers in one or more structures have torn (for instance, a ruptured peroneus brevis tendon that occurs along with ruptured ligaments in a lateral ankle sprain). The affected joint is completely unstable and nonfunctional. Severe pain and massive swelling usually occur immediately. The athlete will often report a snapping or popping sound when the injury occurred. Third-degree injuries must be attended to immediately by trained medical personnel.

3. *Improper support.* Lack of shock absorption and musculoskeletal support puts excess strain on muscles, tendons, and ligaments. Proper protective gear and footwear on suitable playing surfaces help prevent shock- and support-related injuries.

4. *Biomechanical issues.* An athlete's unique structural makeup may put undue stress on specific muscles, tendons, ligaments, and joints. An athlete exhibiting biomechanical imbalances will benefit from being referred to the proper sports medicine professional for treatment or correction.

Treatment of Acute Injuries

All acute injury to muscles, tendons, and ligaments, even if minor, should be addressed promptly to prevent further damage. This will help minimize time off from training and competition and help ensure that the acute injury does not become chronic.

Immediate Care for Acute Injuries

The use of RICE (rest, meaning to stop using the injured area immediately; ice; compression; and elevation) for acute injuries is a well-established practice across the health and fitness professions. It has been hypothesized, although not necessarily proved through research, that the use of RICE minimizes swelling and ischemic tissue damage, thereby minimizing the extent of any hematoma and secondary injury. Traditional thinking is that the injury should be treated with RICE as quickly as possible. The sooner the ice and compression are applied, the more effective they will be in minimizing secondary injury. Ice with compression is typically applied to the affected area immediately for 10 to 15 minutes and every 60 to 90 minutes thereafter to help control the inflammatory response, minimize swelling, limit the spread of secondary injury, and control pain. Elevation of the injured area is also thought to help control swelling via natural gravity flow away from the joint and to facilitate faster healing.

Resting the injured area and appropriate massage therapy will ensure optimal healing of the damaged tissue by preventing the development of weak, inflexible, and painful scar tissue and its subsequent negative effect on athletic performance. After allowing 24 hours for the inflammatory process to fully develop, reassess the area, and refer all second- and third-degree injuries to an appropriate sports medicine professional for further evaluation and treatment before starting massage.

Cryotherapy

Athletes and sports practitioners have used ice, or cryotherapy, to control the pain and inflammation of acute and chronic injuries for generations. There is broad agreement among practitioners that inflammation is a necessary component of the healing process, but excessive or prolonged inflammation may delay or disrupt the completion of the healing process. Cryotherapy has traditionally been used to limit but not eliminate inflammation, as well as to control swelling and reduce pain.

Kenneth Knight, PhD, ATC, published *Cryotherapy in Sport Injury Management* in 1995, and it quickly became the go-to cryotherapy resource for practitioners. He has since written several textbooks for athletic trainers, including one with David O. Draper, *Therapeutic Modalities: The Art and Science, Second Edition,* published in 2013. They include an extensive and well-referenced discussion supporting the proper use of cryotherapy in the treatment of acute, subacute, and chronic injuries.

In recent years, a significant anticryotherapy movement has emerged, arguing that enough research now exists to show that cryotherapy applications delay healing of acute injuries. Gabe Mirkin, MD, is one of the experts who has published commentary against the use of ice. Mirkin takes credit for coining the acronym RICE when he and coauthor Marshall Hoffman published *The Sports Medicine Book* (1978). In 2015, Mirkin walked back his thinking on RICE, especially the use of ice to control inflammation.

Dr. Mirkin refers to a 2004 review of 22 studies that found almost no evidence that ice and compression promoted faster healing. The study authors concluded,

> There was little evidence to suggest that the addition of ice to compression had any significant effect, but this was restricted to treatment of hospital inpatients. Few studies assessed the effectiveness of ice on closed soft tissue injury, and there was no evidence of an optimal mode or duration of treatment. (Bleakley, McDonough, and MacAuley 2004, p. 220)

It's important to note that this review did not find evidence that ice and compression delayed healing.

Two other popular proponents of the no-ice approach for acute injury are Gary Reinl, the author of *Iced! The Illusionary Treatment Option* (2014), and Josh Stone, ATC, CSCS, who has written extensively on his blog on the detrimental effects of cryotherapy for acute injuries (stoneathleticmedicine.com). Both of these authors provide ample research to support their conclusions.

The anti-ice proponents argue that, although ice may provide some pain relief, it delays healing by interrupting the inflammatory process, by interfering with the removal of edema from the injured area, and by preventing or slowing the release of the hormone known as insulin-like growth factor (IGF-1). IGF-1 stimulates cell growth and proliferation and inhibits cell death.

In a 2011 animal-based experiment, the effects of cryotherapy on healing after a skeletal muscle crush injury were studied (Takagi et al.). Immediately following the lab-induced injury, the experimental rats were randomly divided into no-ice and icing groups. In the latter, crushed-ice packs were applied for 20 minutes. The authors then microscopically and physiologically analyzed the healing progression of the injured muscles at 12 hours and then every day for the first 7 days and at 14 and 28 days after the injury. The results of the study showed that "icing applied soon after the injury not only considerably retarded muscle regeneration but also induced impairment of muscle regeneration along with excessive collagen deposition" (Takagi et al. 2011, p. 388). The takeaway from these results is that cryotherapy applied immediately postinjury has both short-term and long-term negative effects on muscle healing. It appears that the temporary pain relief afforded by using ice for 20 minutes creates detrimental effects on the muscle-healing process and may produce weaker and more fibrotic muscle tissue.

A separate study also indicates that icing may produce fibrosis during the healing process (Shibaguchi et al. 2016). The researchers applied ice for 20 minutes to injured rats, then applied heat stress (107°F for 30 min) on the experimental group every other day for the next 14 days. They found that the recovery of muscle mass, protein content, and muscle fiber size toward the levels of the uninjured control group was greater in the heat-stress group and that fibrosis increased in the icing-only group. These findings indicate that using heat on acute injuries, previously anathema, may instead be a viable intervention to promote complete healing of injured skeletal muscles.

As the ice versus no-ice debate continues, practitioners are using several alternative interventions to promote more efficient recovery from acute injury. These may include treatments based on traditional Chinese medicine, or variations on the RICE protocol.

Traditional Chinese Medicine   Traditional Chinese medicine (TCM) has always eschewed the use of ice for treating acute injuries. According to Bisio (2004), TCM sports medicine practitioners believe that cold and damp invades the injured area, congesting and congealing the blood and *qi* (also written as *chi* and meaning vital energy). This stagnation leads to a cascade of effects, including chronic swelling that is hard to disperse and "an arthritic type of pain that often increases with weather changes and is difficult to treat" (Bisio 2004, p. 23). TCM offers several alternative interventions to treat the swelling and inflammation of acute injuries. These include acupuncture, herbal poultices, massage with special liniments, cupping and bleeding, and oral herbal remedies.

POLICE   Bleakley and colleagues (2012) have proposed POLICE (protection, optimal loading, ice, compression, and elevation). According to this editorial,

> POLICE . . . is not simply a formula but a reminder to clinicians to think differently and seek out new and innovative strategies for safe and effective loading in acute soft tissue injury management. Optimal loading is an umbrella term for any mechanotherapy intervention and includes a wide range of manual techniques currently available; indeed, the term may include manual techniques such as massage refined to maximise the mechano-effect... POLICE is not just an acronym to guide management but a stimulus to a new field of research. It is important that this research includes more rigorous examination of the role of ICE in acute injury management. Currently, cold-induced analgesia and the assurance and support provided by compression and elevation are enough to retain ICE within the acronym. (2012, p. 220)

MEAT   MEAT (movement, exercise, analgesia, treatment) has emerged as another alternative to RICE for treating acute soft tissue injuries, especially injuries to tendons and ligaments. The rationale for using MEAT is that early movement and appropriate exercise is better for recovery than immobilization. Buckwalter (1995) discussed the importance of controlled early resumption of activities to promote restoration of ligament and tendon function.

A systematic review of 21 studies was done in 2002 to compare the results of immobilization versus functional treatment for acute lateral ankle sprains. The reviewers concluded that

> Functional treatment appears to be the favourable strategy for treating acute ankle sprains when compared with immobilisation. However, these results should be interpreted with caution, as most of the differences are not significant after exclusion of the low-quality trials. Many trials were poorly reported and there was variety amongst the functional treatments evaluated. (Kerkhoffs et al. 2002, p. 2)

As physicians, sports medicine practitioners, and researchers continue to explore these issues, it's important to remember that while each of these approaches has pros and cons, the quality of the research comparing these interventions leaves a lot to be desired. At this point in the debate, however, it appears safe to assume the cryotherapy portion of RICE is ill-advised, and movement is preferred over immobilization. The challenge for sports massage therapists is to understand, and to help their athletes understand, the rationale for not using ice, especially those athletes with a long history of using ice as their recovery modality of choice.

Chronic Injuries

Chronic injuries to muscles, tendons, and ligaments can be the result of the failed healing of acute injuries or caused by overuse (repetitive microtrauma). According to Shultz and colleagues, "Chronic injury often occurs following periods of inadequate rest or recovery, overuse of a muscle or body part, repetitive overloading of a structure, or repetitive friction between two structures" (Shultz, Houglum, and Perring 2005, p. 7). In many chronic injuries, the underlying cause of pain is often poorly formed scar tissue that interferes with proper muscle strength and contraction or causes poor joint mechanics, or both.

Chronic injuries that result from poorly healed acute injuries (think chronic ankle sprain) may manifest as ligament laxity or muscle weakness that leaves the joint susceptible to acute reinjury or to intermittent exacerbations. In chronic ankle sprain, for instance, ligaments injured in the acute sprain may have never fully healed and will still be tender to palpation, especially at their attachment sites, for years afterward. In addition, the peroneal muscles are commonly strained during an ankle sprain event and may be tender to palpation as well as weak long after the original insult.

In muscle bellies, chronic injuries resulting from an acute strain manifest as dysfunctional scar tissue and may be palpable as a fibrotic area in the affected muscle. The athlete often reports a sense of weakness, that the muscle feels like it's going to cramp, or that it becomes painful at a certain level of activity.

Myotendinous junctions (MTJ) are susceptible to strain or to an overuse injury caused by repetitive microtrauma. Because the MTJ is the transitional area between muscle bellies and tendons, it is subject to high levels of longitudinal strain as well as shearing forces. This may make it susceptible to repetitive microtrauma earlier than either its muscle belly or its tendon. Unfortunately, research evidence about the composition of the MTJ and its adaptability to loading through activity or exercise is lacking.

Overuse injuries in tendons commonly appear as some type of tendinopathy (degradation of the tendon tissue) or tenosynovitis (inflammation of the tendon and its sheath). The athlete typically describes the pain as developing over time, as opposed to the acute injury scenario. In this type of chronic injury, repeated stresses on the tendon create a vicious cycle of inflammation and repair that interferes with the ability of the tissue to properly heal, eventually changing the nature of the tendinous tissue (Zitnay, Li, and Qin, 2017).

Experimental evidence confirms that many chronic tendon injuries, formerly thought to be tendinitis, that is, including inflammation, show degradation of the collagen fibers that make up the tendon with no inflammation present. These conditions are more appropriately called tendinosis or tendinopathy (Bass 2012). See figure 4.2 for a comparison of a normal tendon with tendinitis and tendinosis or tendinopathy.

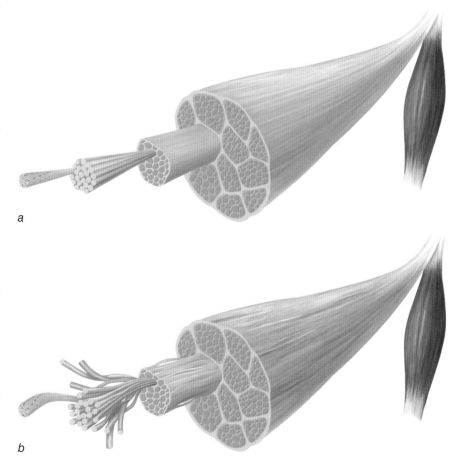

FIGURE 4.2 *(a)* A normal tendon shows intact, bundled collagen fibrils, whereas *(b)* tendinopathy or tendinosis is characterized by disorganized and poorly repaired tendon fibers.

Sports massage techniques, especially friction massage, can be successful in treating chronic soft tissue injuries. In the case of tendinopathy, it appears that the combination of pressure and movement on tendon tissue encourages the fibroblast proliferation needed to remodel the damaged collagen (Lowe 2015). This may also be the mechanism at play in the treatment of scar tissue in muscle bellies and the success of friction massage for treating ligament injuries.

Soft Tissue Injury Repair Process

Because torn muscle tissue has a limited capability to regenerate, healing is accomplished by repair through scar formation. Tendons and ligaments heal initially with scar tissue, but they seem to be able to regenerate over time. Frequently, however, scar tissue ends up as a mass of matted, inelastic fibers that feels thick and fibrous to palpation. If the scar forms improperly, it can render the injured tissue inflexible and irritating to surrounding healthy tissue, creating chronic low-level inflammation, intermittent swelling, and a pain–spasm–pain cycle. If this scarring is not dealt with, any recovery from injury will be temporary because the scar itself is now a source of recurring pain and irritation. However, when an orderly network of healthy collagen fibrils develops, the resulting scar will be strong, pliable, and pain free. This functional scar is developed by ensuring the proper alignment of the scar fibers with one another along the normal lines of stress on the structure. This alignment is accomplished through therapeutic movement and the use of clinical sports massage techniques.

Tissue Healing

Injured soft tissue progresses through a mostly predictable three-phase healing process. Understanding what happens during each of these phases helps the sports massage therapist decide on the appropriate intervention to promote the best outcome during each part of the healing process. The three phases of healing are the inflammatory phase, the proliferative (repair) phase, and the remodeling (maturation) phase (see figure 4.3). Although these phases proceed in order, overlap is significant as one phase ends and the next begins. The typical time line and corresponding characteristics of each of these phases is summarized in table 4.1.

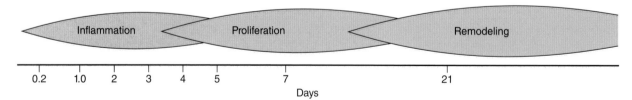

| 0.2 | 1.0 | 2 | 3 | 4 | 5 | 7 | 21 |

Days

FIGURE 4.3   Chronology of tissue healing.

Inflammatory Phase

The inflammatory phase is the body's first line of defense against injury and may last from a few hours to 4 to 5 days. The acute inflammatory response includes immediate vasoconstriction followed by vasodilation, increased permeability of blood vessels, and the migration of fluids, proteins, and white blood cells to the area of tissue damage. The result of increased blood flow and white cell activity create the four

TABLE 4.1 Phases of Healing

Phase	Duration	Characteristics	Goal
Inflammatory	Up to 5 days	At onset of injury, area is warm, red, swollen, and tender.	Stabilize and contain area of injury.
Proliferative (reparative)	Up to 21 days	Scar tissue is red and larger than normal because of edema.	Dispose of dead tissue, mobilize fibroblasts, and restore circulation.
Remodeling	1 year or more	Water content of the scar is reduced; vascularity and redness are reduced; scar tissue density increases.	Stabilize and reestablish the area.

Adapted by permission from S. K. Hillman, *Core Concepts in Athletic Training and Therapy* (Champaign, IL: Human Kinetics, 2012), 373.

cardinal signs of inflammation: redness (Latin *rubor*), heat (*calor*), swelling (*tumor*), and pain (*dolor*). A fifth cardinal sign is the loss of function (*functio laea*) that results from pain with use or swelling that prevents movement (Rather 1971). Although athletes and clients often consider inflammation to be a negative occurrence, it's actually a vital component of the healing process. Without the inflammatory process, the next phases of healing will not occur. Inflammation can become a problem if it does not resolve correctly. If the immune system overreacts to the injury, inflammation can spiral out of control, turning into a chronic inflammatory condition that prevents healing from occurring. Traditional intervention during this phase has been the use of RICE to control swelling and inflammation. Referring back to the earlier discussion of cryotherapy, the current thinking would discourage the use of ice and encourage careful, pain-free movement of the injured area, accompanied by massage techniques such as effleurage to help minimize swelling.

Proliferative Phase

The proliferative, or repair, phase begins as the inflammatory phase is ending. During this proliferative phase, new capillary networks form to facilitate the flow of blood and nutrients into the injured area. Fibroblasts migrate to the injury site and produce collagen to start forming the scar tissue that will eventually replace the damaged tissue. In this stage, the collagenous scar tissue has limited tensile strength and serves merely as a matrix to bind the injured tissue together. This phase may last for several weeks.

During this proliferative phase, pain-free therapeutic movement (active or passive) can be used to help develop a functional scar. However, because the scar lacks tensile strength, stretching should be avoided to prevent tearing the newly forming scar tissue. Because of the wide variations in the severity of soft tissue injuries, no standard exists for how long it takes for a newly forming scar to be able to tolerate stretching beyond normal ROM activity (Orchard 2002). A good rule of thumb to follow in these cases is to wait at least two weeks postinjury before initiating stretching exercises. These should always take place in the pain-free range. During this period, massage using gentle transverse strokes may help the development of normal scarring and discourage the formation of unwanted cross-links or adhesions between layers of fascia.

Remodeling Phase

Remodeling, or maturation, of the initial scar begins as the proliferative phase is ending and may last up to a year or even more. During this phase, the flimsy scar formed during the proliferative phase is slowly rebuilt with stronger, more functional type 1 collagen. The scar fibers develop a parallel orientation along the lines of stress placed on the tissue. Therapeutic movement, combined with sports massage therapy, can be implemented during this phase to help optimize the remodeled tissue.

In some cases, the scar does not remodel properly. According to Mann and colleagues (2011, p. 17),

> Fibrosis is the end result of a complex series of events that follow tissue damage and inflammation. If this process is faulty, excessive and persistent ECM (extra-cellular matrix) deposition takes place, and normal tissue is substituted by collagen scar, resulting in tissue dysfunction.

NERVE ENTRAPMENT CONDITIONS

Sports massage practitioners are often called on to treat chronic conditions resulting from nerve injuries caused by direct pressure on a nerve, commonly referred to as compression or entrapment syndromes. According to Hanna, nerve entrapment syndromes are "disorders of the peripheral nerves that are characterized by pain and/or loss of function (motor and/or sensory) of the nerves as a result of chronic compression" (2017, p. 1). He goes on to assert that "In cases of nerve entrapment, at least one portion of the compressive surfaces is mobile. This results in either a repetitive 'slapping' insult or a 'rubbing/sliding' compression against sharp, tight edges, with motion at the adjacent joint that results in a chronic injury" (2017, p. 2).

Nerve entrapment syndromes develop in a similar fashion to overuse injuries in muscles and tendons. Repetitive microtrauma as a nerve is repeatedly compressed or when a tethered nerve is repetitively stretched at the entrapment site creates a pattern of low-level inflammation and swelling. This, in turn, leads to the development of microfibrosis in and between the fascial layers of the nerve. This fibrosis leads to reductions in the axoplasmic flow.

Axoplasm is the specialized form of cytoplasm found in nerves. Axoplasmic flow (axonal transport) is the process whereby axoplasm, containing proteins and neurotransmitters, flows from the neuron's cell body all along the axon to supply the nourishment and components necessary for the function and repair of the nerve. In chronic nerve entrapment syndromes, axoplasmic flow is compromised, resulting in damage to the nerve axon and the myelin sheath. According to Hanna, "Focal segmental demyelination at the area of compression is a common feature of compression syndromes" (2017, p. 3).

Sports massage techniques can be helpful in treating nerve entrapment syndromes because the soft tissue work helps reduce muscular hypertonicity and improve the ability of fascial layers to move on one another, reducing compressive forces on the nerve and allowing it to slide, not stretch, through its entire pathway (Field, Diego, and Cullen 2004; Elliot and Burkett 2013).

In addition to excessive scar formation, other causes of the failure to completely remodel may be related to improper or inadequate recovery strategies (not allowing enough time for the tissue to recover before going back to sport, aggressive stretching), inadequate nutrition, or extensive immobilization of the injured part. Therefore, the sports massage therapist should be communicating to the athlete the importance of adequate recovery time, optimal nutrition, and therapeutic movement of the injured part, along with the appropriate massage for the tissue-healing phase.

Summary

This chapter has provided an overview of the nature and variety of acute and chronic soft tissue injuries, discussed the classifications used to grade soft tissue injuries, discussed the three stages of healing following a soft tissue injury, and outlined the appropriate sports massage interventions for each. The pros and cons of cryotherapy have been discussed, with the conclusion that the use of ice in treating acute injuries is to be avoided.

Chronic muscle, tendon, and ligament injuries can be successfully treated using specific massage techniques that combine appropriate pressure and friction. Nerve entrapment syndromes are also amenable to treatment using soft tissue interventions to reduce muscle hypertonicity and to alleviate compressive forces on the injured nerve. An understanding of these topics is critical for developing an appropriate injury treatment plan using the sports massage techniques detailed in the following chapters.

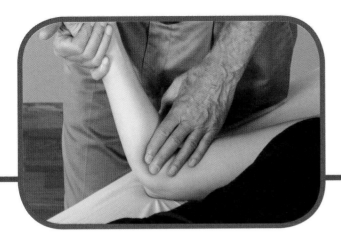

Chapter 5

Soft Tissue Techniques

This chapter discusses and describes sports massage techniques widely used by sports massage therapists to address common musculoskeletal complaints presented by clients. Sports massage practitioners, athletes, and coaches provide a plethora of anecdotal evidence that sports massage is an effective intervention in the treatment of chronic soft tissue injuries and acute injuries that are in the rehabilitation stage. The bulk of peer-reviewed research in this area is inconclusive, but it trends toward support for sports massage for athletic recovery, injury care, and performance enhancement (Crane et al. 2012; Field, Diego, and Hernandez-Reif 2010; Butterfield et al. 2008; Smith et al. 1994). Most professionals decry the paucity of effective studies and advocate for continued research into sports massage using well-designed studies with treatment performed by practitioners specifically trained to administer sports massage therapy.

General sports massage uses the classic Swedish massage strokes: effleurage, petrissage, frictions, tapotement, and jostling. These classic strokes have been adapted by sports massage therapists to help promote injury prevention through optimal recovery from training and as part of an overall strategy when treating injuries. Sports massage also makes use of rhythmic compressions (especially in event work), as well as other myofascial techniques adapted for specific applications. Sports massage typically includes some form of stretching as well. In the context of injury care work, the addition of deep transverse friction, pin-and-stretch methods, and isolytic contractions gives the sports massage practitioner a full range of options for effectively treating soft tissue injuries. Because the training for sports massage is not standardized in the United States (neither in length of training, the way techniques are taught, nor even the terminology used to name the strokes), and because sports massage techniques used outside the United States are sometimes different than those used in the USA, the following discussion of massage strokes is intended to ensure that readers are familiar with the author's use and application of the terms as they apply to sports massage.

Compressive Effleurage

Effleurage is the classical massage stroke thought to stimulate the circulation of blood and lymph. It is a longitudinal stroke along the length of the muscle fibers and generally in the direction of the heart. Superficial effleurage is the stroke commonly used at the beginning of a massage session to apply the massage lubricant and is intended to slightly stretch and stimulate the skin and begin moving blood toward the heart. Effleurage is also used as a transition stroke and has a sedative effect on the nervous system.

Compressive effleurage, as used in sports massage, is a more vigorous stroke than classic effleurage, generally applied using shorter, faster strokes. Compressive effleurage penetrates more deeply than classic effleurage, has a much more profound effect than superficial effleurage, and is intended to be stimulating rather than sedating.

Compressive effleurage is performed with moderate to deep pressure. The practitioner's hands conform to the body part being worked on, and the pressure comes from shifting body weight through the movement of the legs and hips through the arms to the hands (see figure 5.1).

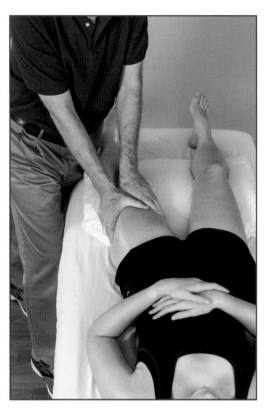

FIGURE 5.1 Compressive effleurage is a preliminary stroke used to warm and stimulate the muscles in preparation for more specific work. Pressure is applied evenly through the palms and fingers.

Compressive Petrissage

Petrissage, or kneading, is another classical massage stroke, generally used after effleurage to continue to warm the muscles, to stimulate the flow of blood and lymph, and to separate layers of tissue. The compressive petrissage used in sports massage is performed as an alternating, kneading stroke that lifts and squeezes muscles and fascia to soften, lengthen, and broaden them. Compressive petrissage is a faster, more vigorous stroke than classic petrissage and uses moderate to deep pressure (see figure 5.2). Because compressive petrissage is directed toward deeper tissues, it's generally preceded by compressive effleurage as the preparatory work. In addition to loosening and softening deeper tissues, compressive petrissage may also have an effect on fluid movement in and through the tissue by reducing restrictions around blood vessels and lymph channels.

To perform compressive petrissage effectively, the practitioner keeps the palms and fingers in full contact with the tissue. This

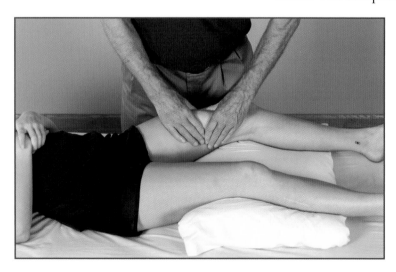

FIGURE 5.2 Compressive petrissage is a brisk, kneading stroke that lifts and separates the muscle tissues.

broad, "soft hand" contact creates less stress in the small muscles of the fingers and feels more comfortable to the athlete than a "pinchy" type of petrissage that occurs when just the fingers are used.

Broad Cross-Fiber Stroke

Broad cross-fiber strokes, also known as muscle broadening or cross-fiber fanning, are administered perpendicularly to the long axis of the muscle and can be administered to just about any muscle, but are especially effective on the larger muscles of the hips, legs, arms, and back. Broad cross-fiber strokes stretch and separate the muscle fibers, with the intention of helping to prevent the formation of adhesions within and between muscles and fascial layers. When bands of muscle fibers feel ropey during muscle broadening, extra attention is given to that section of the muscle belly to restore the ability of the fibers to spread apart.

Various styles of broadening strokes are advocated by different experts. In his classic book, Bob King (1993) describes placing the palms along and parallel to the muscles to be treated, with the thumbs an inch or two (2.5–5 cm) apart (see figure 5.3a). Then, while maintaining pressure on the tissues, the practitioner slowly slides the hands away from each other (see figure 5.3b). The thumbs and thenar eminences provide the delivery of this technique.

Athletic massage specialist and author Pat Archer (2007) credits Benny Vaughn ATC, LMT, for introducing active assistive broadening to the sports massage community. In this style of broadening stroke, the athlete is positioned so that the targeted muscle is in a neutral or lengthened position. The practitioner then places loose fists or heels of hands together at the distal or proximal ends of the muscle (see figure 5.4a). As the athlete slowly contracts the muscle concentrically,

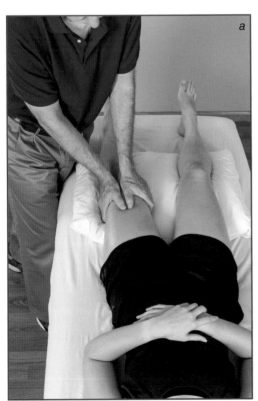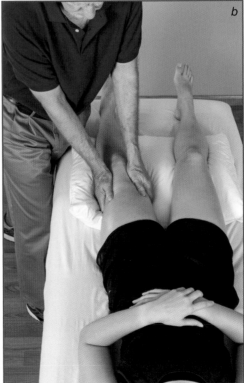

FIGURE 5.3 *(a)* Start the broadening stroke with soft hands and the thumbs slightly apart, and *(b)* maintain moderate pressure on the muscle and slide the hands apart to spread the muscle fibers.

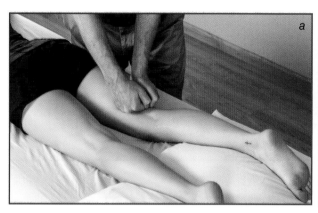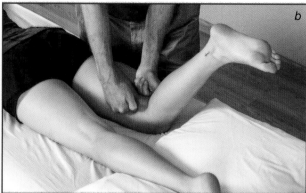

FIGURE 5.4   *(a)* Apply an active assistive broadening stroke by using loose fists to apply moderate pressure and *(b)* then sliding the hands apart as the athlete slowly contracts the hamstrings.

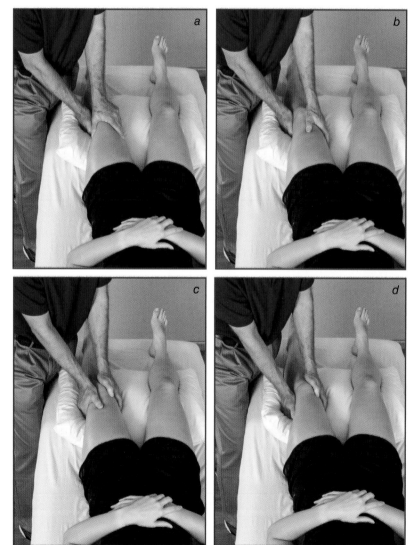

FIGURE 5.5   *(a)* Begin the broad cross-fiber stroke to the relaxed muscle belly and *(b)* fan across the grain of the muscle from lateral to medial. Since the broad cross-fiber stroke is administered in both directions, repeat it in reverse, going from *(c)* medial to *(d)* lateral.

the practitioner applies moderate pressure and slowly slides the hands apart to accentuate the broadening action of the muscle as it shortens (see figure 5.4*b*). This process is repeated until the entire muscle belly has been addressed.

This author prefers the method taught by the late massage educator and author John Harris (Harris and Kenyon 2002), wherein broad cross-fiber strokes are performed across the grain of the relaxed muscle and applied using the thumbs and thenar eminences, flat fingers, or loose fists, with moderate to deep pressure, and using bodyweight and leverage. This is sometimes called a strumming stroke.

The broad cross-fiber stroke is administered slowly enough to allow the muscle fibers to spread under the practitioner's pressure and is performed first in one direction across the entire muscle belly then repeated in the opposite direction across the entire muscle belly. Administering the stroke in this way helps to maximize the beneficial effects of separating the fibers and helps more clearly identify areas of the muscle that are not broadening well. Muscles that are worked in this way function more efficiently because they can shorten and broaden completely during concentric contractions (see figure 5.5).

Longitudinal Stripping

Stripping strokes, administered along the length of the muscle, are effective for deep muscular relaxation. Longitudinal stripping is thought to break up small spasms within the muscle, mildly stretch the muscle fibers longitudinally, and help bring about a lasting hyperemia through deep flushing of the tissues.

Stripping strokes are generally applied with the pads of the thumbs (side by side, one behind the other, or one on top of the other), a loose fist, or the flats of the knuckles (see figure 5.6 for an example of thumbs side by side). The amount of pressure applied will vary with the bulk and density of the muscle being addressed. The client must be as relaxed as possible for this stroke to penetrate deeply without pain.

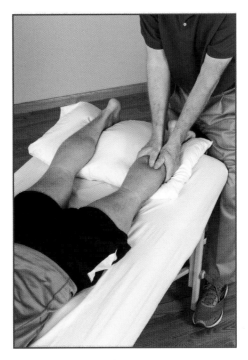

FIGURE 5.6 Stripping strokes performed along the length of the muscle using thumbs side by side.

Case Study

Female Volleyball Player with Back Pain

The client was a 15-year-old female volleyball player (middle hitter/blocker, right handed) complaining of mid-back pain that affected her hitting. A spinal X-ray at age 8 showed scoliosis at the mid-thoracic level. As directed by her doctor, she received massage therapy on a regular basis to keep her muscles pliable in preparation for the teenage growth spurt.

Assessment showed a scoliotic curve to the right with contracted musculature to the left of the spine, tautness on the right, and tightness of the right psoas and high right ilium. Massage therapy treatment consisted of myofascial techniques followed by deep friction to lengthen the left erectors and to release the right latissimus, intercostals, rotator cuff muscles, and trapezius (specifically lower). Kinesiology tape was applied for scoliosis.

This athlete also received physical therapy (postural restoration technique) and was assigned exercises to reduce rotation and strengthen the right psoas. Chiropractic adjustments assisted in aligning the pelvis. Client continued massage therapy twice a week for two weeks. Pain lessened and hitting became easier. I continued to work with the athlete regularly throughout high school. As long as she continued her PT exercises and regular stretching, she only had occasional flare-ups, usually from overuse (hard practices or long games) or long bouts of sitting (studying).

Gay A. Koopman, LMT, BCTMB, CMLDT
Momentum Therapeutic Massage, LLC, Ft Collins, CO

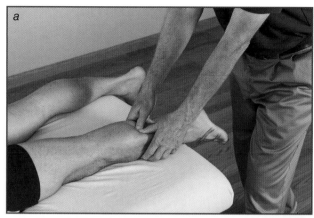

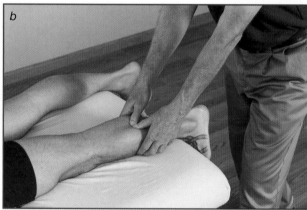

FIGURE 5.7 *(a)* Starting and *(b)* ending position for active pin and stretch of the gastrocnemius.

Pin-and-Stretch Techniques

Pin-and-stretch massage techniques have become popular in recent years through the work of P. Michael Leahy, DC; Whitney Lowe; Joe Muscolino, DC; and others. Archer (2007) refers to this technique as active-assistive lengthening. In the basic protocol, the practitioner applies pressure to selected tissues in the shortened range, then maintains that contact while actively or passively moving the body part from the shortened muscle position to the lengthened position (see figure 5.7).

The rationale for this technique is based on two primary hypotheses:

1. Maintaining a constant, specific pressure on the selected tissue while lengthening it improves tissue function by reducing tissue stiffness, softening fibrosis, and freeing adhesions (Kim, Sung, and Lee 2017).

2. Pressure in the presence of motion may stimulate joint receptors and cutaneous mechanoreceptors to facilitate a "reset" of the autonomic nervous system so the tissue functions more normally (Duncan 2014; Enoka 2015).

Isolytic Contractions

An isolytic contraction is a therapeutically applied eccentric contraction. An eccentric contraction occurs when a muscle is lengthening against resistance. For instance, after performing a dumbbell biceps curl (a concentric contraction), the biceps are contracting eccentrically to control the weight as it's lowered.

Isolytic contractions are used therapeutically because they are thought to break down adhesions or soften fibrotic tissue that may have formed within and between layers of tissues (Chaitow 2001). Isolytic contractions may also "promote orientation of collagen fibers along the lines of stress and direction of movement, limit infiltration of cross bridges between collagen fibers, and prevent excessive collagen formation preventing any muscle stiffness" (Parmar, Shyam, and Sabnis 2011, p. 26). Isolytic contractions make use of modulated levels of eccentric resistance to help improve muscle pliability and function. This technique may be uncomfortable for the client but should remain pain free at all times. The rationale for this technique is that isolytic contractions cause controlled trauma to dysfunctional, fibrotic tissues, while sparing healthy tissue. This is followed by a healing process in which the fibrotic tissue is remodeled with healthier, more functional tissue. In the basic protocol, the muscles to be treated are fully shortened (passively or actively), then the client is asked to resist, but allow, the practitioner's attempt to fully lengthen the muscles. The isolytic contraction lasts 3 to 5 seconds and remains pain free throughout (see figure 5.8).

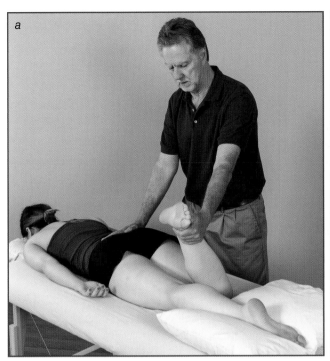
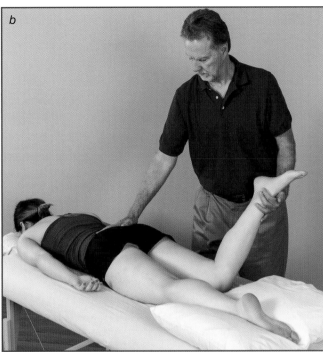

FIGURE 5.8   The isolytic contraction for the hip lateral rotators *(a)* begins with the femur in lateral rotation and *(b)* the practitioner rotates the femur medially as the athlete resists, to lengthen the hip lateral rotators.

Several rounds of isolytic effort are usually required to complete the protocol. In the first round, the client is asked to resist the lengthening motion using 10% to 20% of their maximal effort. In subsequent rounds, the client works harder, even up to maximal effort, as long as the therapist can overcome the effort, and the client remains pain free.

In addition to possibly reducing fibrotic tissue, this technique appears to help reduce protective inhibition and return the treated muscle to full activation.

Deep Transverse Friction

The basis for the deep transverse friction (DTF) treatment described in this section was developed and organized by the late James Cyriax, MD, during his 40 years of research and medical practice and published in his classic book, *Cyriax's Illustrated Manual of Orthopaedic Medicine* (1983). The assessment and deep transverse friction treatment methods he pioneered are an integral component of this author's education and in his ongoing injury care work with athletes. Deep transverse friction is often the missing link in the complete rehabilitation of soft tissue injuries. Unfortunately, many massage therapists have not been trained to use deep transverse friction. To that end, this section delves deeply into the correct application of DTF with the aim of reintroducing it to the field of sports massage for injury care.

As with the broad cross-fiber stroke, deep transverse friction is administered across the grain of the target tissue but is much more site specific than broad cross-fiber work. DTF is generally applied using braced fingers, the thumb, or both. Because the intent of transverse friction is to move and stretch the skin and superficial tissue across the underlying target structures (as if the fingers were glued to the skin), the stroke is administered without lubrication (see figure 5.9). Once the

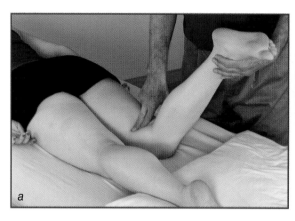 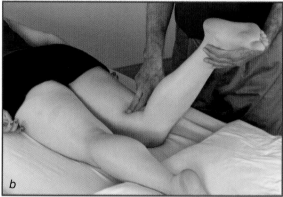

FIGURE 5.9   Deep transverse friction to the distal myotendinous junction of the hamstrings. *(a)* Sink into the tissue to access the tendon and administer the stroke by moving the overlying tissue first in one direction, then *(b)* in the other direction, as far as the skin will stretch.

practitioner has applied adequate pressure to access the lesion, the overlying tissue is moved as a unit back and forth across the lesion as far as the skin will stretch.

General Principles of Transverse Friction

According to Cyriax (1983), deep transverse friction (referred to by others as cross-fiber friction) administered for the treatment of injured muscle bellies, tendons, and ligaments helps realign damaged fibers and soften or eliminate already-formed dysfunctional scar tissue. This in turn reduces the associated inflammation, swelling, and pain.

Modifications to the original Cyriax protocols have been made by practitioners over the years, including those detailed in *Fix Pain* by Harris and Kenyon (2002). The following discussion relies on Cyriax's original work, the work of Harris and Kenyon, and this author's experience.

Transverse friction is an excellent intervention for treating acute, subacute, and chronic muscle and tendon strains and ligament sprains. The intent of transverse friction treatment is to reduce pain, to promote the orderly formation of functional scar tissue by breaking cross-linked adhesions and stimulating increased fibroblast activity, and to encourage more complete healing of soft tissue injuries. The version of deep transverse friction treatments used in this book begin with short sessions, perhaps only a minute, then progress in duration and intensity in subsequent sessions. Assessment is also performed before and after each session to track improvement or lack of improvement and the level of tissue soreness. Modifications to duration and intensity of treatment are then made as necessary. For best results, treatments are given every other day. If this is not possible, then a modified program of self-treatment is developed for the client to perform daily, with weekly appointments with the practitioner to monitor progress and make program changes as appropriate. As a general rule, if deep transverse friction work has not improved the condition within the first three treatments, then a different intervention is called for.

During initial treatment of either acute or chronic injuries, non-weight-bearing and nonresistive ROM help promote the correct alignment of new collagen fibers along the lines of stress on the tissue. According to Harris (2002, p. 47), "Client exercise in the form of non-weight-bearing, non-resisted movement is the easiest way to assist nature in the formation of a pliable, flexible, pain-free scar." Harris goes on to caution that, "Painful adhesions form if weight-bearing exercise, overuse, immobility, or in some cases, stretching or deep massage are initiated too soon."

Archer (2007, p. 159) advocates a slightly different approach to therapeutic movement as part of DTF treatments. She recommends that after DTF applications, the practitioner should "passively move the muscle housing the lesion into a shortened position, then have the athlete perform a minimum of five isometric contractions in this position against manual resistance from the therapist. These isometric contractions serve to enhance the normal muscle-broadening aspect of the injured area. . . . Follow isometric resistives with light stretching." As healing progresses, weight-bearing and resistive exercise may be added cautiously.

Possible Mechanisms of Transverse Friction

Deep transverse friction may stimulate blood flow around tendons and ligaments, promoting the migration of collagen-producing fibroblasts to the injured area. DTF may also increase the secretion of cortisol (a natural anti-inflammatory), promote the release of endogenous pain-relieving substances, and inhibit substance P, a neurotransmitter of pain perception (Harris and Kenyon 2002).

An additional mechanism of action for DTF, based on emerging pain science, has been proposed by science writer (and former massage therapist) Paul Ingraham (2018a, para 26),

> Chronic pain tends to be self-perpetuating. That is, pain can actually make you more sensitive to pain. In a lot of chronic pain cases, the problem is no longer in the tissue, but in nerves that have become oversensitive. Friction massage may interrupt this vicious cycle, by systematically "teaching" the nervous system to be less concerned about stimuli of the irritated tendon. Virtually any stimulation has the potential to do this, but the standard protocol for friction massage might just be particularly good: precisely manageable doses of sensation, repeated over and over again.

Transverse Friction for Assessment and Treatment

Transverse friction techniques may be employed during regular maintenance sports massage sessions to assess the health of tendons, myotendinous junctions, and ligaments. When used for assessment, transverse friction is a moderate-pressure stroke, applied slowly and systematically to the selected tissues. Healthy tissue does not hurt when assessed in this way.

Tenderness in the tissues discovered while applying transverse friction for assessment usually indicates that irritation or an injury process is present, even though the athlete may not be experiencing pain during activity. Harris (2002) refers to this situation as a "prodromal" condition, that is, a subclinical injury, which may lead to an overt injury if left untreated. When used for assessment, transverse friction is administered across the grain of the tissue but in a more general way than when used for treatment. It's generally applied using braced fingers, the thumb, or both. Because the intent with transverse friction is to move and stretch the skin and superficial tissue across the underlying structures (as if the fingers were glued to the skin), the stroke is administered without lubrication.

When pain or tenderness is found during the assessment process, especially if it's prodromal, early intervention and treatment can help improve tissue health before it significantly affects the athlete's performance. Once overt symptoms are present, recovery and rehabilitation will take much longer. Once a dysfunctional scar develops secondary to a soft tissue injury or overuse, efforts to rehabilitate the injury without addressing the scar tissue can be frustratingly ineffective. DTF is often the missing ingredient in the soft tissue injury-rehabilitation process.

Treating Acute Injuries with Transverse Friction

Newly formed scars resulting from strains or sprains are vulnerable to tearing again if stressed incorrectly. All too often, athletes will attempt to rehabilitate their injuries by aggressive stretching and working through the pain. New scars take time to develop enough tensile strength to resist these activities. In the acute stage, injuries respond more favorably to nonresistive and non-weight-bearing movement, giving the scar tissue a favorable environment in which to develop.

In the acute stage of an injury, gentle pain-free transverse friction work can promote the development of adhesion-free scarring by separating and mobilizing potentially adherent collagen fibers to eliminate unwanted cross-links within the scar. This gentle movement also helps to maintain movement between fascial layers. When friction treatments are combined with maintenance sports massage to reduce tension in nearby muscles and with non-weight-bearing ROM activities, the resultant scar will be healthy and resilient.

Treating Chronic Injuries

When scar tissue forms as part of the healing process, the scar frequently ends up as a thickened mass of matted, cross-linked, inelastic fibers that limits pain-free motion and irritates the healthy tissue around it. If this dysfunctional scarring is not dealt with, any recovery from injury will be temporary because the scar itself becomes a source of pain and irritation.

When treating these dysfunctional scars, deep transverse friction is administered to the exact site of the injury. DTF is thought to have a direct mechanical effect on the tissue by abrading the scar. If DTF is administered to the wrong site, little or no therapeutic benefit accrues. DTF can be mildly painful when applied to chronic injuries. Using the 0–10 scale, the therapeutic zone is usually in the range of 6 to 8, as interpreted by the client.

Because the treatment may leave the tissues sore, it is given on alternate days. Treatment is given for only 1 to 2 minutes initially, increasing in duration and intensity as the healing progresses and the formation of functional scarring occurs. The affected area can be iced following treatment to help reduce pain.

Guidelines for Applying Deep Transverse Friction

Because deep transverse friction is a site-specific technique, care must be taken to administer it precisely and efficiently for it to be effective. The primary goal of DTF is to promote the development of properly aligned scar fibers and to reduce unwanted cross-links in the healing tissue. The following six guidelines, originally established by Dr. Cyriax (1983), have since been modified and amended based on clinical experience and anecdotal evidence:

1. DTF is administered to the exact site of the injury. It is thought to create a mechanical effect to soften dysfunctional scarring or to promote the proper

alignment of scar fibers in healing tissue. DTF works only if it's administered to the right place and, if applied incorrectly, may damage healthy tissue.

2. DTF is administered across the grain of the tissue to stretch and separate the fibers in muscle bellies and myotendinous junctions and to abrade the scar in tendons. The stroke must have enough sweep to affect the entire lesion.

3. During DTF, friction (no sliding on the skin) is more important than depth. On a pain scale of 0–10, the therapeutic level is 6 to 8, as determined by the client. In this book, it's understood that above level 8, the client has the urge to pull away, grit his teeth, or hold his breath.

4. Tissue to be treated must be held in the appropriate tension:
   a. *Muscle*. The lesion is often deep in the muscle, so the tissue must be slack in order to reach the fibers to be treated and teased apart. This requires supporting the limb in a way that brings the ends of the muscles toward each other passively.
   b. *Ligament*. The joint is moved to each end of its pain-free range of motion and DTF is applied to the lesion in each position. The goal is to free any adhesions to bone that may be limiting the range of motion of the joint.
   c. *Tendon*: The limb is supported so that the tendon can be held slack or on a stretch, whichever makes it most accessible.
   d. *Sheathed tendon*: Administering DTF with the tendon in a slight stretch allows the tendon to form a solid base that the sheath can be rubbed against, in effect rubbing the scar away.

5. DTF must be administered for the proper duration. Because the treatment is moderately uncomfortable, it's advisable to begin gently and for only 1 to 2 minutes. Treatments are administered every other day because the tissue may be sore the day following a treatment. With each subsequent treatment, increase the DTF time (e.g., 1 minute, 2 minutes, 4 minutes, 6 minutes, up to 10 minutes). Dr. Cyriax recommends 6 to 12 treatments lasting 20 minutes on alternate days. When treating athletes, 8 to 10 minutes of treatment is sufficient and they often heal in 4 to 8 sessions, depending on the severity of the injury.

   Applying ice for 5 to 10 minutes after the treatment will help reduce the soreness until the next treatment.

6. Work cautiously and conscientiously. Refer to a professional when in doubt about the proper course of action.

Facilitated Stretching

Facilitated stretching is an active-assistive stretching technique based on the theories and principles of proprioceptive neuromuscular facilitation (PNF). Elements of PNF are widely used in athletic training rooms, sports medicine clinics, and in personal training (McAtee and Charland 2014). The application of stretching protocols is not appropriate for acute injuries, but it has proven beneficial as part of an overall program of rehabilitation for a variety of soft tissue injuries.

Facilitated stretching falls into a category of stretching called by a variety of names such as muscle energy techniques (MET), active-inhibition techniques, neural-inhibition stretching, and precontraction stretching. These stretching techniques are based on the premise that neurological effects from either isotonic

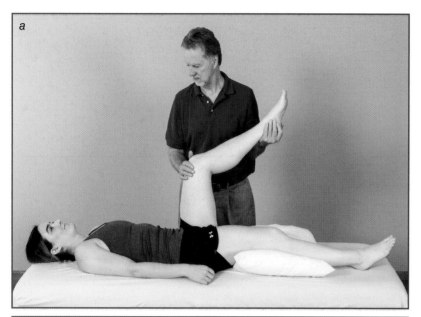

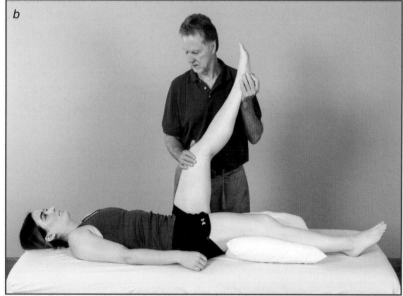

FIGURE 5.10 *(a)* Begin a facilitated stretch for the hamstrings by stabilizing the thigh at 90 degrees of flexion. The athlete isometrically contracts the hamstrings for six seconds by pressing the heel toward the buttock while the practitioner offers matching resistance. *(b)* Following the isometric contraction, the athlete actively extends the knee to stretch the hamstrings to a new ROM without assistance from the practitioner.

or isometric contractions, or both, will inhibit the contractile elements of the target muscle and that this inhibition will dampen resistance to lengthening during the stretch phase.

As described by McAtee and Charland (2014), facilitated stretching uses a combination of *active* movement to the starting point of the stretch, followed by a 6-second isometric contraction of the target muscle to *prepare* it to stretch, then *active* movement to stretch to a new range of motion.

When using facilitated stretching, the sports massage practitioner directs the stretcher to move the limb or body part to the starting position, rather than passively moving the stretcher into position. Following the 6-second isometric contraction, the stretcher actively moves the limb to whatever new range of motion is available without assistance from the practitioner (see figure 5.10).

Summary

This chapter has discussed the sports massage techniques frequently employed to treat common musculoskeletal injuries. In addition to compressive effleurage and petrissage, the use of muscle-broadening strokes and longitudinal stripping are commonly included in the sports massage practitioner's tool kit. Less well-known techniques such as pin and stretch, isolytic contractions, and deep transverse friction are described and discussed in detail to encourage their use in the care and maintenance of injuries. Finally, a brief discussion of facilitated stretching illustrates its use as part of an overall treatment and rehabilitation program.

Part III

Common Neuromuscular Injuries

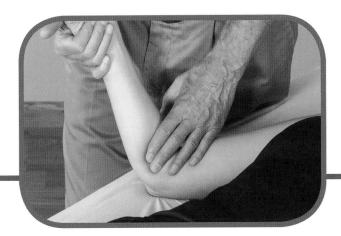

Chapter 6

Treatment of Lower-Extremity Soft Tissue Injuries

Strength, endurance, and flexibility in the hips and legs are critical for success in most sports, especially in those involving running and jumping. Overuse injuries of the lower extremity caused by deficits in strength, endurance, and flexibility are prevalent across the sporting world and affect athletes' ability to train and compete at their highest level.

Sports massage is a beneficial addition to an athlete's training and recovery strategies. Regular maintenance sports massage can aid in the prevention of overuse injuries by monitoring tissue health and making appropriate therapeutic interventions when tissue health is found to be declining. Unfortunately, athletes continue to suffer both acute and chronic injuries, and this chapter presents an in-depth discussion of 10 of the most common injuries assessed and treated by the sports massage practitioner. Admittedly, there are many more soft tissue injuries of the lower extremity that could be included in this chapter, but space considerations have limited the discussion to just these 10. The variety of injuries included here provides a combination of assessment and treatment strategies that can be adapted for use with other sprains, strains, or tendon injuries.

Please note that there are many possible treatment scenarios for the injuries presented here. The suggested treatment progressions for each injury discussed in this chapter are just one treatment option.

Client With Hip Flexor Pain After Hip Replacement

The client is a woman in her mid-60s who complains of complications from hip replacement surgery, causing antalgic gait and pain with active hip flexion. Client had seen multiple orthopedic specialists and completed physical therapy without noticeable improvement in her symptoms. Her goals are to return to physical activity, including strength training and cycling. After recording her history of treatment and discussion and testing of symptoms, it was decided to address her deep hip flexors. These muscles were the target of treatment from the description of symptoms, the expected trauma to these muscles from hip replacement surgery, and the lack of attention to these structures in previous treatment.

The psoas was targeted first, using longitudinal stripping and ischemic pressure with active client hip internal and external rotation. During release of the psoas, she reported pain referral into her anterior hip, consistent with her location of pain. After release of the psoas, she was instructed to walk down the hallway outside the treatment room for feedback on symptoms. She walked without the antalgic gait seen before treatment and reported decreased pain on the hip flexion phase of gait.

Next, the client returned to the table for treatment of the iliacus, using deep transverse friction and treatment of the tensor fasciae latae using broad cross-fiber strokes. On completion of massage techniques, stretching was performed to the hip flexors and TFL. Again, the client was instructed to walk down the hallway for feedback. This time, she broke into a jog halfway down the hallway and returned to the treatment room with a smile on her face. For home care, the client was instructed on proper hip flexor stretching to be performed daily.

She returned for one follow-up 1 week later, reporting improved pain-free hip motion and the ability to ride her bicycle and perform activities of daily living (ADLs). After the follow-up, the client was able to control symptoms with targeted stretching and returned to desired levels of activity.

Earl Wenk, LAT, LMT, ATC, CSCS
Human Performance Collective, LLC, Ann Arbor, Michigan

Achilles tendinopathy is a common overuse injury among athletes participating in racket sports, track and field, volleyball, and soccer. Achilles tendinopathy is also common in endurance runners.

Signs and Symptoms

The typical presentation of Achilles tendinopathy is the gradual onset of pain in the body of the tendon or at its insertion on the calcaneus. Pain may also extend into the foot, creating symptoms similar to plantar fasciitis. In the early stages, pain is often felt at the beginning of a workout, goes away once the tissues are warmed up, and then returns after cool-down. The athlete may also complain of an aching and stiffness in the tendon, especially when arising from sleep or prolonged sitting. This injury may be accompanied by swelling, and in chronic cases, the tendon itself may be thickened. In severe or long-standing cases, there may be one or more tender nodules on the tendon. Crepitus may also be present.

Typical History

Achilles tendinopathy is a perfect example of why it's important to gather a detailed history from an athlete. As with all overuse injuries, Achilles tendinopathy usually develops over a long period, with little or no pain, then may suddenly flare when the athlete increases training activity. For runners, this typically means dramatically increasing mileage or adding speed work or hill running, or all three. Obtaining information from the athlete about their training volume may help pinpoint the reason for a sudden increase in symptoms. Biomechanically, overpronation or a rigid, highly arched foot and a short, tight triceps surae (gastrocnemius and soleus) contribute to the likelihood of developing tendinopathy. In a study of 109 runners with Achilles tendinitis, 40% of the subjects exhibited weakness and lack of flexibility in the triceps surae (Clement 1984).

Relevant Anatomy

The gastrocnemius and soleus muscles form a functional unit called the triceps surae, and they contribute three subtendons to the formation of the Achilles tendon, which just so happens to be the largest tendon in the body. It's been known for many years that the Achilles tendon has a spiral twist of approximately 90° from its origins to its calcaneal insertion (Travell and Simons 1992). For reasons not yet clearly understood, this twist is commonly the most tender portion of an injured Achilles. So it's encouraging that in recent years, anatomical study of the human Achilles tendon has become more detailed. For instance, the orthopedic surgeons who authored a 2014 cadaver dissection study found a consistent "footprint" of the insertion of the Achilles into the calcaneus, reflecting the twist of the subtendons as they approached the calcaneus (Ballal 2014). In their study of 22 human leg specimens, they found that the most superficial aspect of the Achilles is composed of subtendon fibers arising from the medial head of the gastrocnemius that insert along the width of the inferior facet of the calcaneus (see figure 6.1). The deeper part of the Achilles attachment is made up of the soleus subtendon, inserting onto the medial aspect of the middle facet of calcaneus, and the subtendon from the lateral head of the gastrocnemius

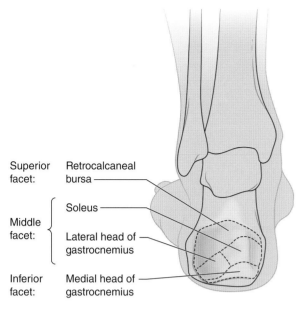

Superior facet:
Retrocalcaneal bursa

Middle facet:
Soleus

Lateral head of gastrocnemius

Inferior facet:
Medial head of gastrocnemius

FIGURE 6.1 The insertional footprint of the subtendons of the triceps surae on the calcaneus.

inserting onto the lateral aspect of the middle facet of the calcaneus.

Researchers from the Jagiellonian University Medical College in Krakow, Poland, investigated specimens of the Achilles tendon still attached to the calcaneus and retaining a fragment of the triceps surae musculature in 53 fresh-frozen male cadavers (n = 106 lower limbs). Their findings support the results of the Ballal study referenced earlier that found that the superficial portion of the Achilles is from the medial head of the gastrocnemius and the deeper portions of the tendon are from the soleus and the lateral head of the gastrocnemius (Pekala 2017). Additionally, these researchers confirmed that as the tendon fibers travel distally toward the insertion, the individual subtendons twist around each other. They also found that the direction of the twist differs, with the left Achilles twisting clockwise and the right Achilles twisting counterclockwise (observing from the superior aspect (myotendinous junction). They identified three distinct types of Achilles tendons (see figure 6.2), based on the amount of twist they exhibit, as follows:

Type I: The least twisted type, found in 52% of the specimens

Type II: Moderately twisted, found in 40% of the specimens

Type III: Extremely twisted, found in 8% of the specimens

This twisting most likely helps provide functional resistance to load stresses on the tendon, but it may also affect the biomechanical properties of the tendon by

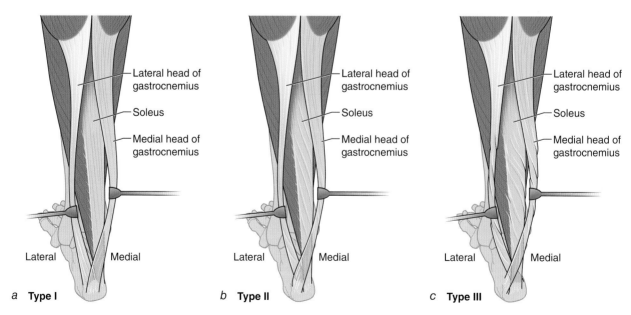

FIGURE 6.2 Three types of Achilles tendon with different degrees of twist in the subtendons: *(a)* type I, *(b)*, type II, and *(c)* type III.

generating an area prone to injury approximately two to three inches (5–7.6 cm) proximal to the insertion (Edama, Kubo, and Onishi 2015).

The Achilles tendon is surrounded by a paratenon, which is similar to a synovial sheath. The paratenon acts as a protective sleeve, which allows gliding motion of the tendon. Dr. Cyriax (1983) theorized that scarring develops on the paratenon as a result of cumulative microtrauma. He taught that this scar tissue then interferes with proper gliding of the tendon, causing irritation and swelling. The injury usually affects the sides and the anterior portion of the tendon, rarely the posterior aspect (see figure 6.3).

More recent research has shown that in painful Achilles tendinopathy, an ingrowth of sensory and sympathetic nerves from the paratenon occurs, resulting in release of nociceptive substances (van Sterkenburg 2011). Interestingly, in a 2015 ultrasound study of the Achilles tendon and paratenon, researchers found a significant correlation between tendon pain and a thickening of the paratenon and theorized that this additional thickness may contribute to the pain of Achilles tendinopathy (Stecco 2015). This thickening is typically palpable in a case of chronic tendinopathy and may be what Cyriax took to be scar tissue.

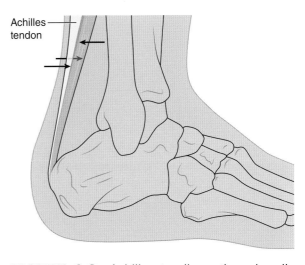

FIGURE 6.3 Achilles tendinopathy primarily affects the medial and lateral aspects of the tendon and often the anterior portion.

Actions and Function

The calf muscles are responsible for plantarflexion of the foot. They also function to provide stability at the foot and ankle. The gastrocnemius also assists knee flexion and is more active in the explosive movements associated with jumping, sprinting, and lifting. A large percentage of fatigue-resistant slow-twitch fibers comprises the soleus, which is more active as a postural muscle in standing, walking, and jogging.

Assessment

Observation

Because Achilles tendinopathy is associated with overpronation or a rigid, highly arched foot, observation of the barefoot athlete walking may reveal the foot on the affected side overpronating or failing to pronate (indicating rigid arch). The tendon on the affected side may exhibit redness, swelling, and thickening of the tendon.

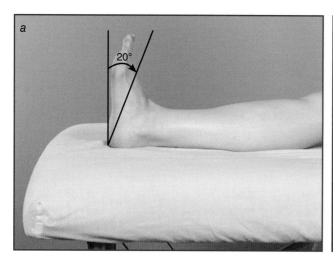

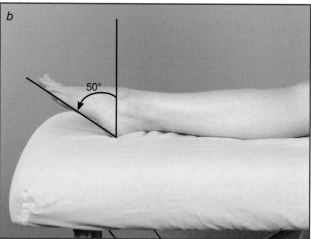

FIGURE 6.4   *(a)* Dorsiflexion is typically 20°. If less than this, shortened calf muscles may be to blame. *(b)* Plantarflexion is typically 50°. A hypertonic anterior tibialis may be the cause of limited range.

ROM Testing

The Achilles tendon is the common tendon of the gastrocnemius and soleus muscles, so ROM assessment includes active, passive, and resisted plantarflexion as well as active and passive dorsiflexion to check for decreased ROM caused by shortened muscles. Normal ROM for dorsiflexion is 20° (see figure 6.4*a*), and normal ROM for plantarflexion is 50° (see figure 6.4*b*). In severe cases, the examiner may hear or feel creaking or crepitus in the tendon during motion.

Manual Resistive Testing

The best muscle test for Achilles tendinopathy is bilateral standing plantarflexion in which the athlete rises onto the toes (see figure 6.5). A positive test reproduces pain. In less severe cases the athlete may need to repeat the test several times on both feet before the tendon pain occurs. If no pain is felt, repeat the test on the affected leg only.

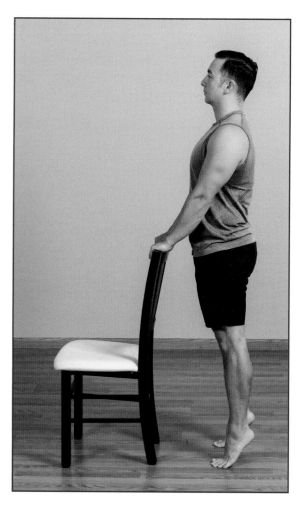

FIGURE 6.5   Bilateral standing plantarflexion.

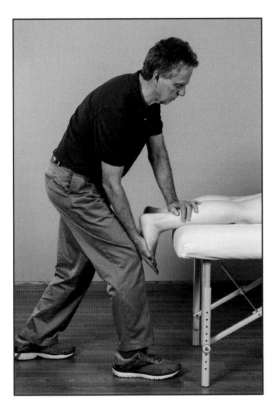

FIGURE 6.6 Resisted plantarflexion.

An additional or alternative test is resisted plantarflexion, where the athlete lies prone on the examination table, with the feet hanging over the edge of the table, ankles relaxed. The practitioner provides graded resistance against the sole of the foot while the athlete isometrically contracts the gastrocnemius and soleus strongly (plantarflexion) (see figure 6.6). Passive dorsiflexion, which stretches the tendon, may also be painful at the end of range.

Palpatory Examination

Palpate the length of the tendon for general thickening, swelling, and tenderness. There may also be one or more tender nodules along the medial or lateral aspects of the tendon.

The Achilles tendon is surrounded by a paratenon and is therefore considered to be a sheathed tendon for purposes of assessment and treatment. Sheathed tendons are best palpated on a slight stretch to provide a firm base to rub the sheath against. Tenderness to palpation may be located anywhere along the tendon, including the myotendinous junction (flat part of the proximal tendon), midtendon, or at the calcaneal insertion (insertional tendinopathy). One side of the tendon may be more tender than the other depending on the factors that contributed to the injury. For instance, an overpronator will generally be more tender on the medial aspect of the tendon.

Differential Diagnosis

Achilles tendinopathy may be accompanied by or mistaken for bursitis, which is an inflammation of one of the bursae at the attachment of the tendon to the calcaneus. The retrocalcaneal bursa is between the calcaneus and the tendon (see figure 6.7); the superficial bursa is between the tendon and the skin. Bursitis is aggravated by massage and responds better when treated with cryotherapy.

To rule out calcaneal bursitis, use the thumb and finger to palpate anterior to the slackened Achilles tendon at its insertion into the calcaneus. Tenderness indicates the possible presence of retrocalcaneal bursitis. Superficial calcaneal bursitis will be painful on the posterior aspect of the Achilles tendon at the calcaneus and may be accompanied by swelling and thickening of the skin.

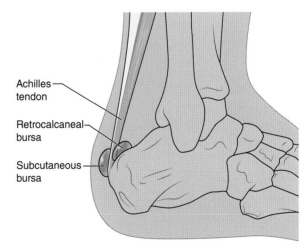

Achilles tendon
Retrocalcaneal bursa
Subcutaneous bursa

FIGURE 6.7 Retrocalcaneal bursae.

Perpetuating Factors

Perpetuating factors must be addressed to prevent the recurrence of the injury. If the condition is the result of excessive pronation of the foot on the affected side, custom orthotics may be necessary. Pelvic imbalance, leg-length discrepancy, and muscle strength and length problems need to be corrected. Training factors that contribute to this condition include running too many miles, excessive hill running (up and down), improper stretching and warm-up, and dancing en pointe. Biomechanical factors affecting this injury include overpronation, a rigid high arch, and hypertonic hamstrings or calf muscles, or both. Equipment-related factors may include shoes that are worn out, or have too much or too little motion control, shoes with inflexible soles, shoes with a stiff heel counter that rubs against the tendon, or shoes with a soft heel counter that fails to stabilize the heel and foot.

Treatment Plan

Deep transverse friction (DTF) is the primary treatment for Achilles tendinopathy. The severity of the problem and the length of time it has been present are both factors that influence recovery.

A typical treatment session is as follows:

1. Administer compressive effleurage and petrissage and broad cross-fiber strokes to the entire lower leg for general warm-up and to reduce the hypertonicity of the gastrocnemius and soleus muscles. Follow with longitudinal stripping to the calf.

2. Administer facilitated stretching of the calf muscles. Stretching combined with the warm-up massage helps further reduce hypertonicity and eases the tension on the Achilles tendon.

3. With the athlete prone, flex the knee and dorsiflex the foot slightly to put a stretch on the affected Achilles tendon. Avoid stretching the tendon so far that the sides cannot be palpated easily. Maintain the stretch by supporting the foot against the practitioner, and use the pads of the thumbs or fingers to palpate the one or two most tender spots on the tendon. Apply DTF by using a rolling motion to and fro, as if rolling a pencil between the thumbs and fingers (see figure 6.8).

The initial application of DTF lasts about 1 minute using moderate pressure, that is, enough pressure to engage the paratenon and roll it against the tendon surface. This may be somewhat painful for the athlete at the beginning, so the practitioner should adjust the

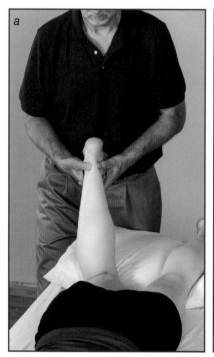
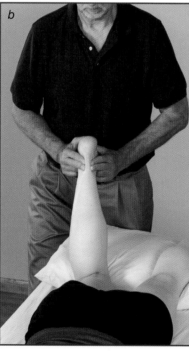

FIGURE 6.8 Administer deep transverse friction (DTF) to the slightly stretched Achilles tendon using the *(a)* thumbs or *(b)* fingers.

pressure to keep the discomfort at about a 6 on a 10-point pain scale. Near the end of the first minute, the discomfort typically will have abated significantly. In some cases, it will remain the same, or it may increase.

Because tendinopathy can also affect the anterior surface of the tendon, it must be treated as well. To make it accessible, passively plantarflex the foot to slacken the tendon, and forcefully push the tendon medially with the thumb. Use braced fingers of the treating hand to apply friction to the anterior surface of the tendon. Keep the finger, hand, and forearm in a straight line with the elbow bent, and apply friction by supinating and pronating the forearm, which rotates the braced finger to and fro against the anterior aspect of the tendon (see figure 6.9). Switch hands and repeat the process by pushing the slackened tendon laterally to access the other part of the anterior tendon.

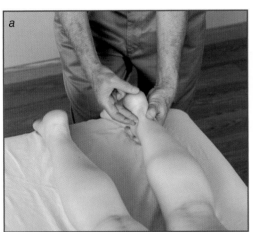 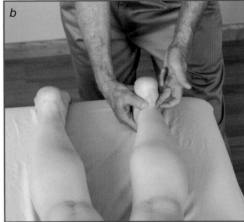

FIGURE 6.9 DTF with braced finger to the anterior portion of the Achilles. *(a)* Treating the medial aspect and *(b)* treating the lateral aspect.

4. After the first minute of DTF, the focus shifts to more general massage for the lower leg, or perhaps to the uninvolved side, to give time for the treated tendon to rest.

5. Return to the affected area for another round of DTF. This time, the duration of treatment may be up to 3 minutes, as long as the discomfort rating is at or below a 6 on a 10-point scale.

6. Administer pain-free isolytic contractions to help reduce protective inhibition and assist the muscles to return to full activation.

7. Finish the treatment with another round of facilitated stretching for the calf muscles.

8. Frequent applications of ice are important to help control pain posttreatment.

9. Ideally, treatment is given every other day. Following the initial session, the friction portion of subsequent sessions can be longer (up to 9 minutes total) but still given in two or three doses per session. Each dose is given long enough for the pain to subside to near zero.

10. The duration of treatment depends on the severity of the injury, the frequency of treatment, and the athlete's self-care activities.

Self-Care Options

If perpetuating factors are noted, these must be modified or eliminated to ensure that the injury does not reoccur. Once the tendon pain is eliminated, initiate a program of flexibility and progressive strengthening. Swimming, pool running, and easy cycling are good alternative exercises for maintaining fitness while reducing stress on the tendon. The athlete should not run again until she can do calf raises without pain. When the athlete is pain free, strengthening the gastrocnemius and soleus can begin. Start with non-weight-bearing, nonresistive repetitions of plantarflexion, and then progress to resistive or weight-bearing activities, or both. These can include seated and standing calf raises, jumping rope, and cycling. Stretching should focus on both the gastrocnemius and the soleus, as well as the hamstrings.

Case Study

Runner With Chronic Achilles Tendinosis

This client is a 57-year-old male middle-distance runner. He initially injured his left Achilles tendon at the 1984 Olympic Trials. It was diagnosed as a grade 2 tear. He was in a boot for 6 weeks but did not receive surgery. He also has a history of rolling the same ankle many times since. His current injury was to the same left Achilles tendon. He noticed pain beginning as the trail running season started. He experienced swelling, redness, and pain around the lower one-third of the tendon, with a defined thickening above the calcaneus. He had been diagnosed with tendinosis by a physical therapist after examination and imaging. This diagnosis required a long-term team approach for a successful outcome that returned the client to running. Once per week the physical therapist performed fairly aggressive instrument-assisted soft tissue mobilization (IASTM) and prescribed eccentric exercises to strengthen the tendon. This was accompanied by soft tissue work once a week.

Because the physical therapy was introducing inflammation by using IASTM and eccentric exercise, the soft tissue work was aimed at two things: managing pain and inflammation and keeping the repairing tissue pliable throughout the healing process. Because the area to be worked was painful to the touch, massage started with gliding effleurage to introduce blood flow and stretch the soft tissue of the lower leg. Reducing tension in the lower leg by slow, deep compression helped to decrease muscle tone. Petrissage was then used around the affected area to help increase viscosity of the healing tissue. Lastly, a pin-and-stretch shearing force was applied directly to the acute area with active movement of the ankle into dorsiflexion and plantarflexion to keep the tendon sheath and tendon from binding.

Treatment outcome was successful with regular weekly massage treatments. The client slowly returned to a walk–run combination and eventually full running.

Molly Verschingel, LMT
Time Out Sports Massage, Tigard, Oregon

It's often been said that it's better to break an ankle than to sprain it. This is because broken ankles are treated as serious injuries and ankle sprains are often treated minimally, if at all. Ankle sprains fall into two broad categories: acute and chronic. Acute sprains happen suddenly. They can be minor or severe and need to be treated appropriately. Unfortunately, many athletes ignore a minor sprain and are prone to "just walk it off" and keep training. Acute sprains not properly cared for become chronic sprains, typically characterized by weakness and hypermobility at the injury site that subjects the ankle to repeated exacerbations.

Signs and Symptoms

The signs and symptoms of an acute inversion sprain (lateral ankle) are pain or tenderness at the injury site; swelling or bruising or both; muscle spasm of the muscles of the foot and leg, especially the fibularis group; and sometimes, a cold foot or paresthesia indicating possible neurovascular injury. The signs and symptoms of a chronic sprain are ongoing low-level pain or tenderness at the injury site; chronic low-level swelling; laxity or instability, where the ankle easily "gives way" during routine activity; and early-onset osteoarthritis of the ankle.

Typical History

Most ankle sprains occur on the lateral ankle from sudden rolling or twisting of the foot, usually including both plantarflexion and inversion, causing an inversion injury. Inversion sprains may involve a stretching or tearing injury to the anterior and posterior talofibular ligaments, the calcaneofibular ligament, and the dorsal calcaneocuboid ligament (see figure 6.10). Grade 1 sprains are normally mild enough to be treated by sports massage therapists without physician clearance. Grades 2 and 3 sprains should be immediately referred to a physician or sports medicine professional.

Once an athlete has experienced an acute ankle sprain, that ankle is more easily sprained again, leading to a chronic sprain condition accompanied by laxity in the ligaments and weakness in the fibularis muscles. There may also be pain with certain movements.

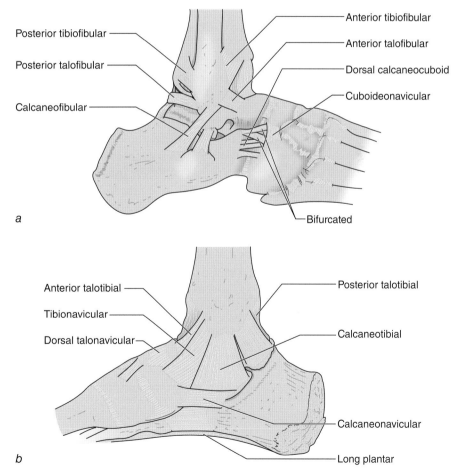

FIGURE 6.10 Ligaments of the (a) lateral ankle and (b) medial ankle.

Relevant Anatomy

The ankle and foot are home to multiple ligaments. The ligaments around the ankle are commonly grouped, based on their position, as the lateral ligaments, the deltoid ligament (medial), and the tibiofibular syndesmosis (stabilizes the tibia and fibula).

The focus in this discussion is on the main lateral ankle ligaments that are subject to injury (see figure 6.11). These include the anterior talofibular ligament (ATFL), the calcaneofibular ligament (CFL), the posterior talofibular ligament (PTFL), and the dorsal calcaneocuboid ligament (DCL).

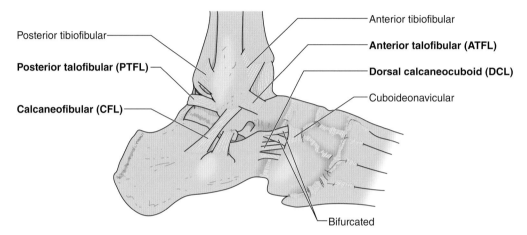

FIGURE 6.11 Lateral ankle ligaments. Names in bold indicate common injury sites in lateral ankle sprain.

The anterior talofibular ligament (ATFL) is the most commonly injured ligament in an inversion sprain. According to Kumai and colleagues (2002), approximately two-thirds of ankle sprains are isolated injuries to the ATFL because it is the weakest ligament in the lateral ankle. This ligament runs nearly horizontal when the ankle is in neutral, slackens in dorsiflexion, and is taut in plantarflexion, making it vulnerable to injury when the foot is forcefully plantarflexed and inverted. The injury typically occurs first at the fibular origin, but a more severe sprain will also injure the talar insertion.

The calcaneofibular ligament (CFL) is the next most commonly injured ligament, even in a grade 1 sprain. When the ankle is in neutral, the CFL angles inferior and slightly posterior from its attachment on the tip of the fibula to the posterior region of the lateral calcaneus. A forceful inversion of the ankle with the foot in neutral or dorsiflexed will injure the CFL, first at the fibular attachment and then at the calcaneus.

The posterior talofibular ligament (PTFL) arises from the posterior aspect of the distal fibula and runs posteriorly to attach to the lateral tubercle on the posterior aspect of the talus. It plays a secondary role in stabilizing the ankle joint and is the least commonly injured of the three ligaments because it is usually subject to sprain only when the foot is fully dorsiflexed.

In addition, the dorsal calcaneocuboid ligament (DCL) is included in this discussion because it is frequently injured in a grade 1 sprain. The DCL, not to be confused with the calcaneocuboid part of the bifurcated ligament, is a thin broad ligament that connects the anterior dorsal aspect of the calcaneus to the dorsal aspect of the cuboid bone. Its position on the foot places it under stress when the foot is plantarflexed. The DCL is thought to be injured in 5% to 6% of all inversion sprains (Lohrer et al. 2006).

It's important to remember that one or more of the peroneal (fibularis) group is likely to suffer a strain injury in an acute lateral ankle sprain. The forceful inversion of the foot overpowers the ability of the fibularis group to resist the motion; therefore, they may sustain a grade 1, or even a grade 2 strain, especially the fibularis brevis.

Assessment

Acute Sprain

The athlete's report of the injury event and the location of pain forms the basis for assessment.

Observation

Look for signs of swelling and bruising at the lateral ankle, sometimes settled by gravity at the inferior aspect of the foot or radiating into the toes. Feel for temperature, especially noting whether the foot is cold because this may indicate neurovascular injury.

ROM Testing

Test pain-free active and passive ROM, with a focus on plantarflexion and inversion. Swelling and pain may prevent normal movement. Note location of pain as reported by the athlete.

Manual Resistive Testing

Resisted tests of the fibularis group may reveal pain and weakness, indicating a strain injury to the muscle bellies or the tendons.

Palpatory Examination

The palpation exam is conducted carefully to locate the most painful areas, indicating the primary injury sites. Because the ATFL is the most commonly injured ligament, careful palpation of the bony attachments will often reveal sharp, pinpoint pain. Palpate the muscles of the foot and leg, especially the fibularis group, to check for swelling, spasm, and pain.

Chronic Sprain

The athlete's report of the original injury event coupled with the ongoing dysfunction (pain, weakness, instability) forms the basis for assessment.

Observation

Chronic sprains often exhibit low-level swelling long after the original injury, especially in cases of recurrent sprains.

ROM Testing

Test pain-free active and passive ROM of the foot and ankle, with a focus on plantarflexion and inversion. Note location of pain as reported by the athlete. Although chronic sprain typically results in joint laxity, in some cases scar tissue from poorly healed ligaments limits ROM. Passive inversion or plantarflexion is often painful because of ligamentous adhesions to the calcaneus or surrounding tissues.

Manual Resistive Testing

Resisted tests of the fibularis group may reveal pain and weakness, indicating an ongoing and untreated strain injury to the muscle bellies or the tendons. Passive inversion may cause pain from stretching injured muscle or tendon tissue or because of adhesions between injured ligaments and the underlying bones or the surrounding soft tissues.

Palpatory Examination

The palpation exam is conducted carefully to locate the most painful areas in each of the suspected ligaments, indicating the ongoing injury sites. Because the ATFL is the most commonly injured ligament, careful palpation of the bony attachments will often reveal low-level pain. Palpate the muscles of the foot and leg, especially the fibularis group for spasm, fibrosis, tenderness, or atrophy.

Precautions and Contraindications

Avoid stretching freshly injured tissues.

Differential Diagnosis

Ankle fracture, talar dome fracture, and rupture of the Achilles or fibularis tendon.

Perpetuating Factors

Perpetuating factors must be addressed to prevent the recurrence of the injury. Pelvic imbalance, leg-length discrepancy, and muscle strength and length problems need to be corrected. Also, incomplete rehabilitation of the sprained ankle leads to instability, weakness, and pain. These factors must be addressed if restoration of normal function is to occur. Training factors that contribute to this condition include improper stretching and warm-up and lack of strength training for the foot and ankle complex. Biomechanical factors affecting this injury include previous ankle sprains, excessive inversion, foot and ankle hypermobility, and muscle strength and length issue in the lower leg and foot. Equipment-related factors may include shoes that are worn out, or have too much or too little motion control, shoes with inflexible soles, shoes with a stiff heel counter that rubs against the tendon, or shoes with a soft heel counter that fails to stabilize the heel and foot.

Treatment Plan

Acute sprains of any severity can benefit from sports massage treatment. Once an ankle sprain becomes chronic, adhesions have likely formed and deep transverse friction is the method of choice for eliminating them.

Treatment of Acute Injury

After physician clearance for grades 2 and 3 sprains and 24 hours after grade 1 sprains, gentle, pain-free effleurage may be administered to help reduce swelling around the ankle. As the swelling and inflammation subside (24–72 hours), gentle, pain-free transverse friction may be added to stimulate proper scar formation in the injured ligaments and to prevent adhesions from forming. As healing progresses (swelling and inflammation are gone), transverse friction may be done more firmly, but remaining pain free. The athlete should continue to support the ankle when bearing weight and maintain active, non-weight-bearing motion of the ankle, including circumduction.

Treatment of Chronic Injury

Based on the probability that scar tissue and adhesions have developed as a result of the original sprain, deep transverse friction is applied to the most tender sites as identified through assessment and palpation. A typical treatment session is as follows:

1. Administer compressive effleurage and petrissage and broad cross-fiber strokes to the entire lower leg for general warm-up and to reduce the hypertonicity of the gastrocnemius, soleus, tibialis anterior, and fibularis muscles.

2. Administer facilitated stretching of the tibialis anterior and fibularis muscles. Stretching combined with the warm-up massage helps further reduce hypertonicity and improve movement of the foot and ankle complex.

3. Based on the findings of the assessment, apply DTF to the affected ligaments. The friction treatment is applied to the injury site with the ligament first held in the slackened position then in the tautened position (see figures 6.12–6.14). Because the ligaments are fairly superficial, minimal pressure is needed to engage the tissue. DTF is administered using the finger pad of a braced finger or the thumb.

    The initial application of DTF lasts 30 to 60 seconds using moderate pressure, that is, enough pressure to engage the ligament against the underlying bone. This may be somewhat painful for the athlete at the beginning, and the practitioner should adjust the pressure to keep the discomfort at about a 6 on a 10-point pain scale. Near the end of the session, the discomfort typically will have abated significantly. In some cases, it will remain the same, or it may increase.

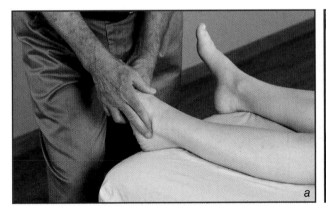 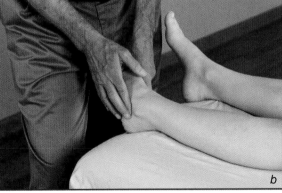

FIGURE 6.12 DTF for the anterior talofibular ligament (ATFL). *(a)* Hold the foot in slight plantarflexion and eversion to slacken the ligament. Braced fingers administer DTF across the ligament at the distal fibula. *(b)* Hold the foot in plantarflexion and inversion to tauten the ligament at its talar attachment. Braced fingers apply DTF across the ligament attachment on the distal fibula.

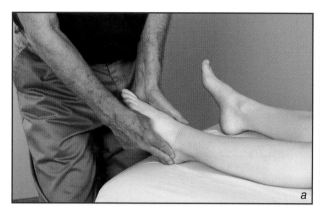
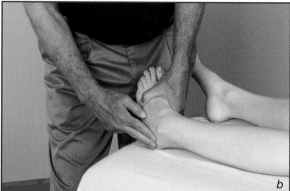

FIGURE 6.13 DTF for the calcaneofibular ligament (CFL). *(a)* Hold the foot in slight eversion to slacken the ligament. Braced fingers administer DTF across the ligament attachment on the distal fibula. *(b)* Hold the foot in inversion to tauten the ligament at its calcaneal attachment. Braced fingers apply DTF across the ligament attachment on the distal fibula.

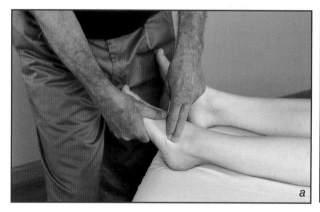
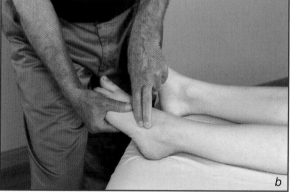

FIGURE 6.14 DTF for the dorsal calcaneocuboid ligament (DCL). This is a short ligament and can be treated with two fingers side by side. *(a)* Hold the foot in neutral to slacken the ligament and administer friction. *(b)* Hold the foot in plantarflexion with forefoot medially rotated to tauten the ligament and administer friction.

4. After the first round of DTF, the focus shifts to more general massage for the lower leg, or perhaps to the uninvolved side, to give time for the treated ligament to rest.

5. Return to the affected area for another round of DTF. This time, the duration of treatment may last up to 3 minutes, as long as the discomfort rating is at or below a 6 on a 10-point scale.

6. Finish the treatment with another round of facilitated stretching for the fibularis group and the tibialis anterior.

7. Ideally, treatment is given every other day. Following the initial session, the friction portion of subsequent sessions can be longer (up to 9 minutes total) but still given in two or three doses per session. Each dose is given long enough for the pain to subside to near zero.

8. The total duration of treatment depends on the severity of the injury, the frequency of treatment, and the athlete's self-care activities.

Self-Care Options

If perpetuating factors are noted, these must be modified or eliminated to ensure that the injury does not reoccur. Swimming, pool running, and easy cycling are good alternative exercises for maintaining fitness while reducing stress on the ankle. Additional components of self-care include strengthening exercises for the tibialis anterior and the fibularis group. Once bearing weight is pain free, balance exercises will stimulate the proprioceptive network that protects the ankle from inversion sprain. Balance work can be accomplished by standing on one foot, standing on one foot with eyes closed, and using a balance beam or a half-ball balance trainer.

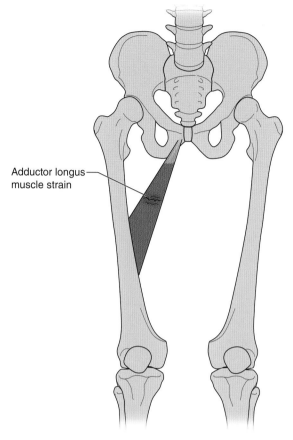

Adductor longus muscle strain

FIGURE 6.15 Groin strain of the adductor longus.

A groin "pull" is a strain to any one of the five adductor muscles: pectineus, adductor brevis, adductor longus, adductor magnus, and gracilis. An adductor strain injury occurs when the tension generated in the adductors exceeds their failure tolerance. Adductor longus is the most commonly injured of the adductor group. This is likely due to its lack of mechanical advantage when the femur is abducted (see figure 6.15).

The exact incidence of adductor muscle strains in most sports is unknown because athletes often play through minor groin pain, and the injury goes unreported. Overlapping diagnoses can also affect the incidences of reported groin strain. In 2010, Tyler and colleagues reported a study of 26 National Hockey League teams that found the incidence of adductor strains increased from 2003 to 2009 and the rate of injury was greatest during the preseason compared to regular and postseason play. In professional hockey and soccer players throughout the world, 10% to 11% of all reported injuries are groin strains. These injuries have been linked to hip muscle weakness, a previous injury to that area, preseason practice sessions, and level of experience (Tyler, Silvers, and Gerhardt 2010).

Signs and Symptoms

Pain in the groin region is the most common symptom of an adductor strain, especially when adducting the legs or flexing the hip on the affected side. Stretching the adductor group may also cause pain at the injury site. Groin strain can be a sudden, acute injury, or it can manifest as an overuse injury that develops over several months, typically resulting in tendinopathy. Chronic groin strain can also be the result of the failed healing of an acute injury, where scar tissue in the muscle belly or the myotendinous junction area perpetuates symptoms. In an acute injury, the athlete may have heard or felt a pop, followed by immediate pain. Depending on severity, acute injury may be accompanied by swelling and bruising along the inner thigh. Acute groin injuries are typically localized at the myotendinous junction of the affected muscles. In overuse groin conditions, pain tends to be more specific to the tendinous attachments on the pubic bone. Chronic groin injuries will be located at the site of the original injury; therefore, they can be found in the muscle belly, the myotendinous junction, or at the tendinous attachments.

Typical History

Groin strains are common in sports that require running, jumping, and quick changes of direction or acceleration, such as soccer or hockey. In ice hockey, groin injuries are common because the diagonal stride used in skating puts the groin muscles under eccentric strain. Overstretching and the eccentric force generated by the adductors as they work to decelerate the limb during rapid abduction and external rotation (as occurs in ice-skating) or a sudden change in direction are all factors that can lead to tension in the tissues that exceeds their failure tolerance. In soccer players, groin strains can be the result of rapid changes of speed and direction or from reaching to the side to acquire the ball. Trail runners are at risk for groin injuries because of the hazards of navigating uneven terrain. Martial artists can incur a groin strain when performing high kicks if they have not fully warmed up or when they're fatigued.

The number one risk factor for sustaining a groin injury is having had a previous groin injury. Many experts attribute this to the incomplete rehabilitation of the original injury, thereby leaving the adductor group weak and inflexible. Poor flexibility is a factor in adductor strains because reduced ROM in hip abduction and hip internal rotation places additional longitudinal and rotational stress on the adductor group during skating, kicking, and running activities. A strength imbalance between the adductor and abductor is a major predisposing factor in groin stains. Adduction strength should be equal to or greater than 80% of abduction. Tyler and colleagues (2002) assessed the adduction-to-abduction strength ratio of 58 professional ice hockey players. Players who had strength ratios less than 80% were considered at risk.

Relevant Anatomy

As previously noted, the adductor group consists of five muscles (see figure 6.16). They all originate from a relatively small area on the pubic bone (except for a portion of the adductor magnus) and fan out to insert along the posteromedial femur (except for the gracilis, whose attachment is on the tibia). Some anatomy teachers use the mnemonic phrase "grab my leg baby, please" to help students remember the adductor muscles from distal to proximal: *g*racilis, adductor *m*agnus, adductor *l*ongus, adductor *b*revis, and *p*ectineus.

Actions and Function

The primary functions of the adductor group include adduction of the thigh in open-chain motions (e.g., kicking a soccer ball or swinging the leg); assistance in internal rotation (which is why aggressive external rotation of the hip can create an adductor strain); deceleration of the lower extremity at the end of abduction and extension, as in skating; and stabilization of the lower extremity and pelvis during weight-bearing. The adductors may generate significant tension in closed-chain activities while attempting to stabilize the hip and control the alignment of the lower limb.

Individually, the gracilis can assist flexion of the thigh or the knee. The adductor magnus (specifically the posterior head) is considered to be a fourth hamstring because, like the hamstrings, it attaches across the ischial tuberosity, is innervated by the sciatic nerve, not the obturator nerve, and can extend the thigh at the hip joint.

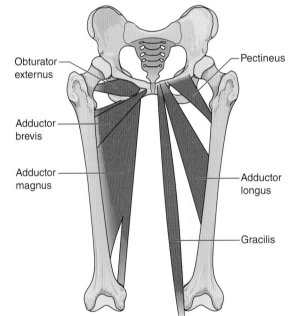

FIGURE 6.16 Adductor group: pectineus, adductor brevis, adductor longus, adductor magnus, and gracilis.

Assessment

Observation

Athletes with acute groin strain typically have a great deal of discomfort with regular adduction (and sometimes abduction) movements, especially those that also include hip flexion, like getting in and out of a car, stair climbing, and putting on socks. Acute strain may also exhibit diffuse bruising. Chronic adductor strain exhibits many of the same symptoms, just at a lower level of intensity and often described as a dull aching pain that is diffuse and hard to pinpoint.

ROM Testing

Active and passive ROM testing is conducted to determine the limits of pain-free motion. In addition to testing single-plane hip flexion, extension, adduction, abduction, and internal and external rotation, it may be necessary to examine triplanar movement through the FABER test (hip *fl*exion, *ab*duction, and *e*xternal *r*otation combined) to pinpoint the location of the pain.

Manual Resistive Testing

If acute groin strain injuries are too painful for even minimal examination, conduct functional muscle testing carefully to avoid causing pain. Always test the unaffected side first. The exact location of a chronic groin injury (either in the muscle belly, the myotendinous junction, or an attachment site) can often be pinpointed using resisted muscle tests.

The most common muscle test for groin strain is resisted single-leg adduction in several positions (leg straight, knee and hip flexed, slight abduction, and external rotation). Varying the test position can help pinpoint the pain location. See figure 6.17 for an example of two test positions.

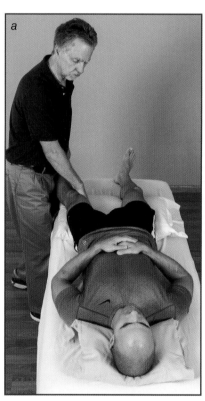 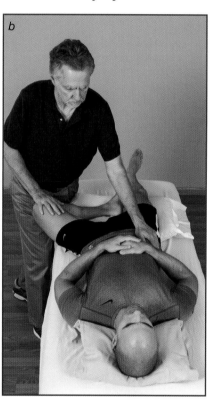

FIGURE 6.17   *(a)* Resisted adduction with the leg straight and *(b)* the FABER test with hip and knee flexion, abduction, external rotation.

Palpatory Examination

For both acute and chronic groin strain, palpation reveals pain in the affected tissues. Although the athlete can often point to the exact site of pain, palpation is conducted throughout the adductor group, including the pubic attachments (with informed consent) to determine the exact location of the lesion.

Precautions and Contraindications

Avoid direct pressure over the femoral artery, vein, and nerve as they pass through the femoral triangle. Some acute groin strains are accompanied by swelling and ecchymosis. Avoid deep massage until these conditions resolve.

Differential Diagnosis

Although diagnosing acute groin strain is usually fairly straightforward, chronic groin issues can be quite challenging. According to Alomar (2015, p. 1),

> Chronic groin pain in particular can be difficult to diagnose, treat, and rehabilitate, and is responsible for a large proportion of time lost from sport and work for the athlete. A complicating component in the treatment of this condition is an extensive differential diagnosis and overlap in symptoms between possible diagnoses.

The main conditions that also present with groin pain include sports hernia, femoroacetabular impingement (FAI), osteitis pubis, and hip labral tear.

Perpetuating Factors

Research has documented that the primary risk factor for a groin strain injury is a previous injury. This is likely caused by incomplete rehabilitation in the past, and this issue must be addressed fully to help prevent a future occurrence. Transverse friction massage helps resolve scar tissue issues in previously injured muscles. But more needs to be addressed. The resolution of pain is not a valid indicator that the athlete is ready to return to play. As noted previously, muscle imbalances play a key role in groin injury. A comprehensive strength and flexibility plan is needed to reduce or eliminate perpetuating factors.

Treatment Plan

The main component of treatment for this condition is transverse friction to the area where pain has been identified through testing and palpation. The most common muscle involved in adductor strain is the adductor longus and the treatment location is typically 2 inches (5 cm) distal to its attachment on the pubic bone. Friction work is best performed in small doses, several times during a session, with two or three sessions per week if possible. Acute cases of adductor strain can benefit from light transverse friction work (see figure 6.18) included as part of an overall massage treatment plan. Avoid massage while bruising is present. In acute cases, the friction work is gently administered with flat fingers across the injured tissue to spread and separate muscle fibers thereby discouraging the development of cross-links and adhesions within the healing tissues.

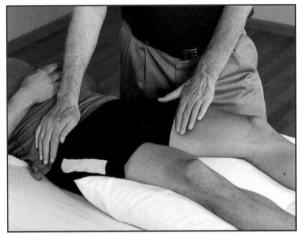

FIGURE 6.18 Light DTF for acute adductor strain using flat fingers.

Chronic groin strain may be the result of an acute injury that has not healed fully or may be an overuse condition brought on by repetitive microtrauma. The dysfunctional tissue may be in the muscle belly, at the myotendinous junction, or at the attachment site of the tendon. For chronic injuries, deep transverse friction is used to help the body normalize tissue quality. Depending on the location of the lesion, DTF may be administered using flat fingers, the thumb, or a pincer grip, as in the description that follows. A typical treatment session for chronic adductor strain in the muscle belly of the adductor longus follows:

1. Administer compressive effleurage and petrissage to the entire lower limb for general warm-up and to reduce the hypertonicity of the surrounding tissues.

2. Administer facilitated stretching of the quadriceps, hip adductor, and hip abductor muscles. Stretching combined with the warm-up massage helps further reduce hypertonicity and eases the tension on the affected muscles.

3. Position the athlete in a comfortable supine position on the treatment table, with a bolster under the knee to allow pain-free hip flexion and abduction, making the adductor longus accessible.

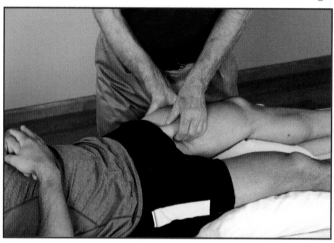

FIGURE 6.19   Moderate DTF for chronic adductor strain using a pincer grip.

4. Use a pincer grip (thumb and index and middle finger) to carefully grasp the adductor longus approximately 2 inches (5 cm) distal to its pubic attachment. Administer moderate-pressure transverse friction by maintaining the pincer position and drawing the hand back and forth across the muscle belly (see figure 6.19).

5. The initial application of DTF lasts about 1 minute using moderate pressure, that is, enough pressure to engage the tissue and "scrub" it transversely. This may be somewhat painful for the athlete at the beginning, so the practitioner should adjust the pressure to keep the discomfort at about a 6 on a 10-point pain scale. Near the end of the first minute, the discomfort typically will have abated significantly. In some cases, it will remain the same, or it may increase.

6. At this point, the treatment shifts back to more general massage for the entire lower extremity, or perhaps to the uninvolved side, to give time for the treated tissue to rest.

7. Return to the adductor longus for another round of DTF. This time, the duration of treatment may be up to 3 minutes, as long as the discomfort rating is at or below a 6 on a 10-point scale.

8. Administer pain-free isolytic contractions to help reduce protective inhibition and help the muscles return to full activation.

9. Finish the treatment with another round of facilitated stretching for the adductor group.

10. Frequent applications of ice are important to help control pain posttreatment.

11. Ideally, treatment is given every other day. Following the initial session, the friction portion of subsequent sessions can be longer (up to 9 minutes total) but still given in two or three doses per session. Each dose is given long enough for the pain to subside to near zero.

12. The total duration of treatment depends on the severity of the injury, the frequency of treatment, and the athlete's self-care activities.

Self-Care Options

If perpetuating factors are noted, they must be modified or eliminated to reduce the likelihood of reinjury. Once the groin pain is eliminated, initiate a program of progressive stretching and strengthening.

Because limited flexibility is associated with acute and chronic groin strain, the athlete should consider a self-care program that includes dynamic warm-ups before activity and facilitated stretching to improve ROM in hip abduction, hip flexion, and internal and external rotation. Because strength imbalances are associated with acute and chronic groin strain, initiating a program to correct them is crucial to minimizing the risk of another injury. According to Tyler and colleagues (2010), a professional hockey player is 17 times more likely to sustain an adductor muscle strain if his adductor strength is less than 80% of his abductor strength. Strength exercises that focus on concentric work, such as ball squeezes, and full-range adduction exercises (seated, side lying) are helpful in developing adductor strength.

An emphasis on eccentric training is important because eccentric muscle contractions train the deceleration function of the adductors. Examples of eccentric-focused exercises include adduction while standing using a cable-pulley machine or elastic resistance and PNF spiral-diagonal leg patterns using a cable-pulley machine or elastic resistance.

Hamstring Tendinopathy

Chronic hamstring tendinopathy is a common running injury that develops over a period of up to 3 months with few or no symptoms. Then pain may suddenly appear as a result of increased athletic intensity such as adding speed work or hill running to a training regimen.

Signs and Symptoms

The condition usually manifests as pain at the proximal myotendinous junction of the hamstring, at the ischial tuberosity, or both. The athlete may complain of achy pain just below the gluteal fold, exacerbated by sitting.

Typical History

Chronic tendinopathy is an overuse injury that typically has a gradual onset of pain, appearing from 6 weeks to as long as 3 months after the onset of the offending activity as degenerative changes develop in the tendon. Athletes with mild to moderate symptoms frequently continue to train, expecting they can run through the pain. In the early stages of this condition, the pain is mild at the beginning of a workout and then goes away once the athlete has fully warmed up. If the injury is not addressed, it slowly progresses to hurting longer at the beginning of a workout and returning at the end after cool-down. Athletes who ignore the early signs of tendinopathy and continue to push past the pain will likely contribute to the development of a more severe and problematic condition that will take much longer to resolve.

Relevant Anatomy

The hamstring muscle group (see figure 6.20) consists of the biceps femoris (long and short head), the semimembranosus, and the semitendinosus. The proximal attachment of the hamstring is the ischial tuberosity (sit bone). The tendons of the biceps femoris and semitendinosus attach to the posteromedial aspect of the ischium and blend with fibers of the sacrotuberous ligament, which in turn attaches to the lateral inferior sacrum (see figure 6.21). The semimembranosus originates from the posterolateral ischial tuberosity, is deep to the semitendinosus and biceps femoris, and is superficial to the horizontal fibers of adductor magnus.

Actions and Function

The hamstring is the primary knee flexor and assists the gluteus maximus with extension of the hip. The biceps femoris laterally rotates the tibia when the knee is bent to 90°, and the semitendinosus and semimembranosus medially rotate the tibia when the knee is bent to 90°.

During walking, running, and jumping activities, the hamstrings contract eccentrically to decelerate hip flexion and knee extension to control the forward motion of the leg as it approaches ground contact. They also function eccentrically to stabilize the knee and counteract rotational forces when landing with a bent knee.

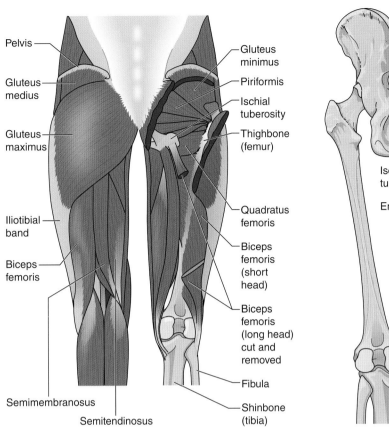

FIGURE 6.20 Hamstring muscle group.

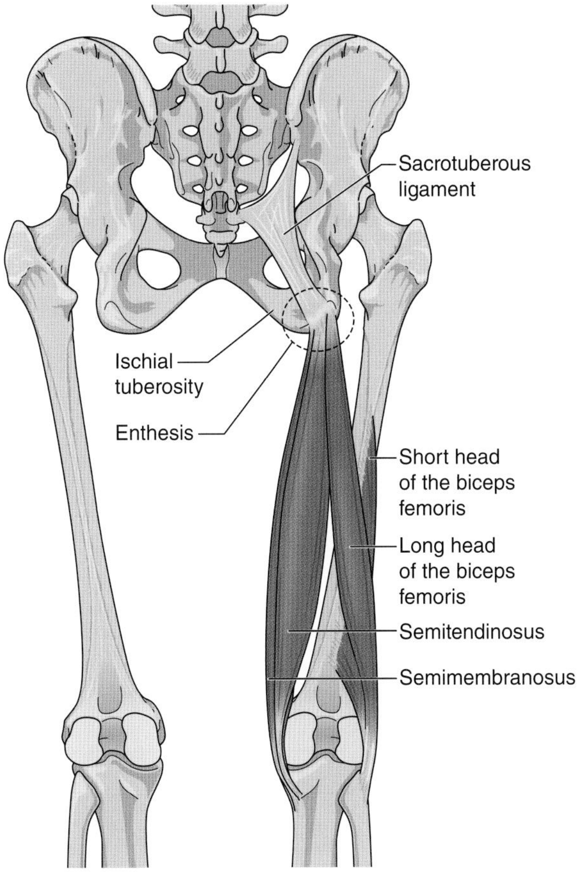

FIGURE 6.21 Ischial attachments of the hamstring blending with the sacrotuberous ligament.

Assessment

Observation

Chronic hamstring tendinopathy is most commonly located at the attachment site on the ischial tuberosity. Pain may also be reported just distal to the origin, indicating an injury at the myotendinous junction of the biceps femoris. If the athlete is not complaining of symptoms, but the pain in the tissue is felt during a maintenance sports massage, the following assessments may not isolate the problem area because the condition is not advanced. If the athlete is already complaining of symptoms, these tests should be, but are not always, positive.

ROM Testing

Hypertonicity in the bilateral hamstrings, quadriceps, and iliopsoas interacts with bony imbalances to create conditions for tendinopathy to develop. Pain may be felt during passive hamstring stretching, either as a straight-leg test or during knee extension with the hip flexed to 90°.

Manual Resistive Testing

These tests for hamstring injury are considered positive if they re-create the athlete's pain or reveal weakness or if the muscle belly begins to cramp:

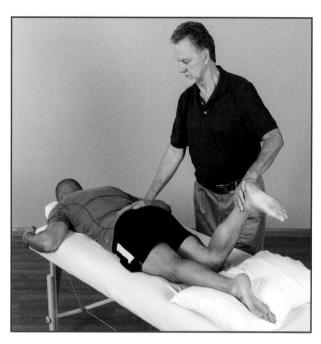

FIGURE 6.22   Resisted knee flexion test.

Resisted Knee Flexion

With the client prone, the knee of the affected leg is flexed to approximately 90°. The practitioner stabilizes the hip and leg with one hand and provides resistance at the client's heel with the other. The client then slowly contracts the hamstrings isometrically (knee flexion), increasing the strength of the contraction incrementally to maximal (see figure 6.22). If pain or cramping occurs, end the test.

If desired, the practitioner can further isolate the hamstring muscles by rotation of the tibia on the bent knee: Engage the medial hamstring more effectively by laterally rotating the tibia on the femur so that the heel points toward the midline (see figure 6.23a). Engage the lateral hamstring more effectively by medially rotating the tibia on the femur so that the heel points away from the midline (see figure 6.23b).

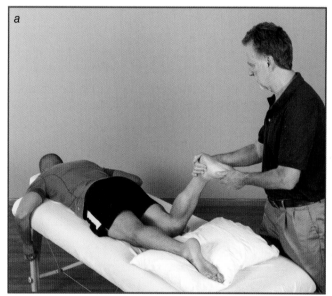
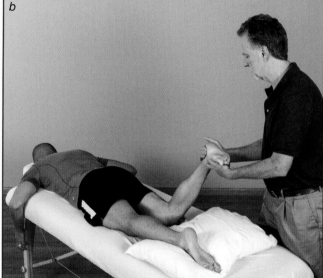

FIGURE 6.23   Further isolating (a) the medial hamstring and (b) the lateral hamstring in the resisted knee flexion test.

Resisted Hip Extension

With the client prone, the knee of the affected leg is flexed to approximately 90°. The practitioner places a hand at the distal thigh to provide resistance as the client slowly contracts the hamstring (and gluteus maximus) isometrically, attempting to extend the hip. The client's effort increases incrementally to maximal (see figure 6.24). If pain or cramping occurs, end the test.

If any of these tests are positive, the practitioner then palpates to determine the exact site of the lesion in the area where the athlete reported the pain. Tests that do not re-create the pain indicate a low-level injury, and it is still worthwhile to palpate the hamstring tissues to search for lesions that might be the source of the complaint.

Palpatory Examination

Hamstring tendinopathy is far more common at the origin or at the proximal myotendinous junction than at the insertion. Pain on palpation indicates that an active injury process is present. If the origin is tender, the myotendinous junction will almost always be tender as well. The palpation exam should assess for tenderness in the sacrotuberous ligament because it is, in effect, an extension of the origin of the biceps femoris and the semitendinosus. Frequently, the sacrotuberous ligament is the site of the lesion and the ischial tuberosity will be pain free during palpation.

Accurate palpation of the hamstring origin on the ischial tuberosity can be accomplished through a variety of positions. Remember, the tendons are wide as well as thick. With the athlete prone and ankles bolstered to slacken the hamstrings, use the pads of the fingers to palpate the ischial tuberosity. Use moderate pressure to press the tendons against the tuberosity and apply a cross-fiber stroke, relying on the athlete to report the most tender area. The cross-fiber stroke must have enough sweep to palpate the entire width of the origin (see figure 6.25). For a deeper lesion, it's necessary to bring the deep semimembranosus tendon closer to the surface to palpate it effectively. The athlete is in a side-lying position, with the affected leg on top and the knee and hip flexed and relaxed. Apply the friction stroke by standing in front of the athlete and reaching across the body to the ischial tuberosity (see figure 6.26). This position enables the use of body weight to apply the stroke.

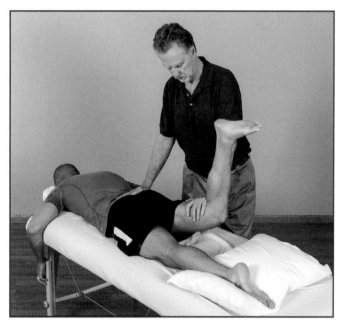

FIGURE 6.24 Resisted hip extension test.

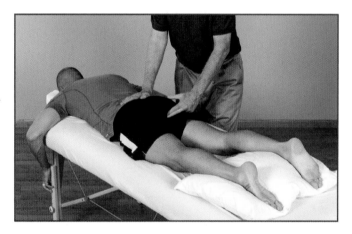

FIGURE 6.25 Palpation of the hamstring at its origin.

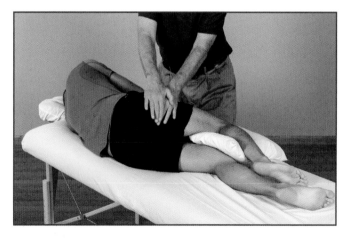

FIGURE 6.26 Palpation of the semimembranosus tendon of the hamstring.

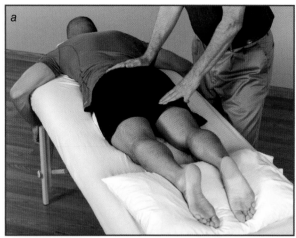

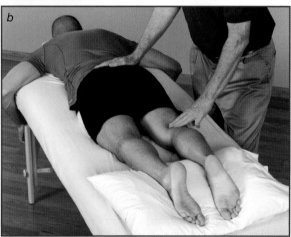

FIGURE 6.27 Palpation of the *(a)* proximal and *(b)* distal myotendinous junctions of the hamstrings.

The palpatory exam at the myotendinous junctions is performed by applying moderate downward pressure with the flats of the fingers to the suspected area then moving in a cross-fiber direction to assess for pain (see figure 6.27). Because of the width of the tissue at this point, it may be necessary to work in several strips.

Precautions and Contraindications

Because the friction work may sometimes be administered close to the athlete's groin area, fair warning should be given and informed consent should be obtained before treatment.

Differential Diagnosis

Sciatic nerve pain, piriformis syndrome, and ischiogluteal bursitis.

Perpetuating Factors

Hamstring tendinopathy is highly correlated with overuse. Factors include training too much or at too high an intensity. A runner may be shifting from long, slow distance to speed work or hill running. Proper stretching and warm-up may be lacking. Biomechanical factors include pelvic imbalances, leg-length differences, imbalances in muscle strength or length or both (shortened quadriceps and weak, tight hamstrings), and overstriding in running that may perpetuate or aggravate hamstring tendinopathy. The hamstrings and gluteals may not be contracting in the proper sequence. Equipment issues that may contribute to this condition include worn or broken-down running shoes, poorly fitting orthotics, and improper fit on the bike.

Treatment Plan

Deep transverse friction is extremely effective in treating hamstring tendinopathy. Friction work is best performed in small doses several times during a session, with two or three sessions per week if possible. When treated this way, even long-standing tendinopathy responds favorably in a relatively short time.

A typical treatment session is as follows:

1. Administer compressive effleurage and petrissage to the entire lower limb for general warm-up and to reduce the hypertonicity of the surrounding tissues.

2. Administer facilitated stretching of the hamstrings and calf muscles. Stretching combined with the warm-up massage helps further reduce hypertonicity and eases the tension on the tendon.

3. To treat the ischial tuberosity, the athlete is prone and ankles bolstered to slacken the hamstrings. Use the pads of the fingers to palpate the ischial tuberosity as shown in figure 6.25. Use moderate pressure to press

the tendons against the tuberosity and apply a transverse friction stroke, relying on the athlete to report the most tender area. The transverse stroke must have enough sweep to palpate the entire width of the tendinous attachment. The initial application of DTF lasts about 1 minute using moderate pressure, that is, enough pressure to engage the tissue and "scrub" it against the bone. This may be somewhat painful for the athlete at the beginning, so the practitioner should adjust the pressure to keep the discomfort at about a 6 on a 10-point pain scale. Near the end of the first minute, the discomfort typically will have abated significantly. In some cases, it will remain the same, or it may increase.

4. For a deeper lesion, it's necessary to bring the deep semimembranosus tendon closer to the surface to palpate and treat it effectively, as shown in figure 6.26. The athlete is in a side-lying position, with the affected leg on top and the knee and hip flexed and relaxed. Apply the transverse friction stroke with braced fingers by standing in front of the athlete and reaching across the body to the ischial tuberosity. Maintain moderate pressure on the tuberosity, keep the arms straight, and rock forward and backward from a lunge stance, thereby using body weight and good mechanics to administer the treatment.

5. Treat the myotendinous junctions by applying DTF using the flats of the fingers to apply moderate downward pressure on the suspected area and then moving in a transverse direction to treat the lesion as shown in figure 6.27. Because of the width of the tissue at this point, it may be necessary to work in several strips.

6. After the first minute of DTF, the focus shifts to more general massage for the entire lower extremity, or perhaps to the uninvolved side, to give time for the treated tendon to rest.

7. Return to the affected area for another round of DTF. This time, the duration of treatment may be up to 3 minutes, as long as the discomfort rating is at or below a 6 on a 10-point scale.

8. Administer pain-free isolytic contractions to help reduce protective inhibition and help the muscles return to full activation.

9. Finish the treatment with another round of facilitated stretching for the hamstring and calf muscles.

10. Frequent applications of ice are important to help control pain post-treatment.

11. Ideally, treatment is given every other day. Following the initial session, the friction portion of subsequent sessions can be longer (up to 9 minutes total) but still given in two or three doses per session. Each dose is given long enough for the pain to subside to near zero.

12. The total duration of treatment depends on the severity of the injury, the frequency of treatment, and the athlete's self-care activities.

Self-Care Options

If perpetuating factors are noted, these must be modified or eliminated to ensure that the injury does not reoccur. Once the tendon pain is eliminated, a program of flexibility and progressive strengthening can be initiated. Hamstring injuries of all types indicate a need to assess the strength ratio between the hamstrings and quadriceps. Pelvic imbalances can also create undue tensile stress on the hamstrings, causing them to be stretched and tight simultaneously. Once these imbalances are corrected, begin a program of facilitated stretching for the hamstrings, calf muscles, quadriceps, and hip flexors.

Therapeutic eccentric exercise is the currently accepted first choice for helping rehabilitate tendinopathy. According to Cushman and Rho (2015, p. 3), "The beneficial effects of eccentric exercises have been attributed to the greater tendon load generated when compared to concentric exercises, increased collagen synthesis, decreased neovascularization, and force fluctuations from tendon loading and unloading."

Triathlete With Right Hamstring Injury

Client is a 42-year-old male triathlete. During a training ride on his road bike he was hit by a slow-moving car. He rolled over the hood of the car and landed on the ground. No major injuries occurred, but he stated his right outside, posterior knee was sore. He continued to train (swim, run, bike) but stated his right leg didn't feel right. Right hip, hamstring, and calf felt "congested and tight." He stated he felt a clicking sensation in his right knee when running and biking. (He rated his pain at 2 on a scale of 10). Even though he didn't injure his right calf, he noticed that it would cramp during his swim and bike sessions.

On evaluation, the distal, lateral right hamstring exhibited mild irritation with knee extension but not knee flexion. Assisted straight-leg raise with the left leg was 90°, with no pain and moderate stretch. Assisted straight-leg raise with the right leg was 80°, with mild tightness and no pain. Palpation over the distal biceps femoris elicited mild pain. Assessment was mild right distal hamstring strain.

Treatment focused on the full right leg from the glutes to the calf. Treatment started with manual work over the gluteus maximus and gluteus medius to decrease guarding in the glute complex. This was followed by right hip rotations in a prone position with bent knee. Internal and external rotation pin and stretch was performed. Manual work of compression, stripping, and pin and stretch was applied to the hamstring complex but with focus over the biceps femoris. IASTM was performed at the distal biceps femoris over the musculotendinous junction. Cupping with silicone cups was applied and actively moved by the therapist up and down the entire hamstring complex.

When this work was done, the therapist applied assisted stretching while the client was supine on the table. This was applied in multiple angles moving from straight up to diagonal across the body, eliciting a stretch over different fibers of the hamstring complex. When the client was in a supine position with a straight leg across his body in a stretch position, the therapist positioned the leg and created a pin and stretch with the biceps femoris musculotendinous junction with an active knee flexion and extension movement. Finally, the therapist did manual work (compression, petrissage, stripping) over the right calf and finished with cupping work with therapist-assisted movement over the calf.

The injury didn't stop the athlete from working out, but it did hamper his performance, and he found it annoying. Because he planned to ramp up his training for future Ironman competitions, he feared that this injury would get worse. The athlete continued to work with his training coach and came in for weekly sessions for about 6 weeks. The right hamstring was the primary concern, and other body treatments were secondary. The coach and the therapist continued to talk over the 6 weeks exchanging notes and progress. If the coach noted that a movement pattern of the athlete's right leg was off, the therapist would address it in treatment sessions. The therapist also informed the coach of the type of treatment performed and advised altering the workout for that day to help with recovery. By the end of the 6 weeks, the athlete's hamstring flexibility was equal to that of his noninjured leg; he felt no pain with palpation over the distal biceps femoris, and cramping in his right calf ceased.

This treatment was a success, and the athlete is now performing with no pain in his hamstring. The coach and therapist continue to keep in contact while both work with this athlete as he continues to train for the Ironman World Championships in Kona, Hawaii.

Delaney Farmer, LAT, LMT, ATC
PRM Sports Therapy, Bellevue, Washington

Iliotibial Band Syndrome

Iliotibial band syndrome (ITBS) is an overuse injury characterized by pain felt at either the insertion of the IT band at Gerdy's tubercle (lateral proximal tibia) or just proximal to the lateral femoral condyle or both. ITBS occurs commonly in novice runners with overpronation problems, but it can affect runners at every level of accomplishment. It also occurs frequently in cyclists, soccer players, rowing athletes, and hikers. Tautness in the IT band can be the result of hypertonicity in the tensor fasciae latae and gluteus maximus or from hypertrophy of the vastus lateralis, which bulges under the band and places excessive tensile stress on it, or both.

Although IT band syndrome has traditionally been considered a friction syndrome, where the band rubs across the lateral femoral epicondyle during knee flexion and extension, new evidence supports a different causation. In 2007, Fairclough and colleagues published an in-depth study of the IT band anatomy, specifically looking for evidence that it rubbed or rolled across the lateral femoral epicondyle. Their findings show that the IT band, a thickening of the fascia lata that surrounds the thigh, firmly attaches via an intermuscular septum all along the linea aspera of the femur. Distally, the IT band attaches to the femoral condyle and epicondyle by coarse fibrous bands (sometimes mistakenly identified during palpation for dysfunctional adhesions), attaches to Gerdy's tubercle on the lateral tibia, and connects fascially to the lateral patella. The authors assert that these anatomical attachments preclude the IT band from moving back and forth across the epicondyle and that the pain of IT band syndrome is the result of the compression of a richly innervated and vascularized fat pad that lies between the IT band and the femoral condyle. Fairclough concluded that "ITB syndrome is related to impaired function of hip and leg musculature and its resolution can only be achieved through proper restoration of lower quadrant muscle balance" (Fairclough et al. 2007, p. 74). Based on these findings and other anatomical and biomechanics research, Geisler and Lazenby (2017) suggest renaming the condition iliotibial band impingement syndrome (ITBIS) to reflect the newer evidence-informed assessment and treatment of the condition.

Signs and Symptoms

Athletes typically present with tenderness just proximal to the lateral femoral epicondyle or at the proximal lateral tibia (Gerdy's tubercle) and report a sharp, burning pain when they press on the lateral epicondyle during knee flexion and extension (see figure 6.28). The pain is particularly acute when the knee is at 30° of flexion.

Typical History

As with all overuse injuries, the onset of pain associated with ITBS is gradual, worsening over time as the athlete continues to train. Pain often subsides when the athlete modifies or suspends training, only to return when the training intensifies.

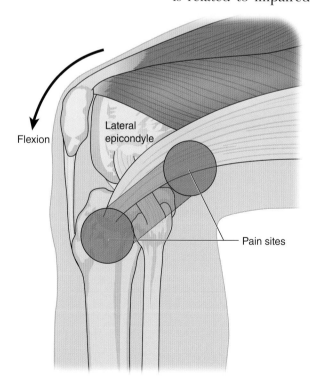

FIGURE 6.28 Typical IT band injury sites.

Flexion

Lateral epicondyle

Pain sites

Relevant Anatomy

The IT band is a fibrous thickening of the lateral aspect of the fascia lata, a fascial sleeve that surrounds the thigh musculature like a stocking. Part of the fascia lata originates from the anterolateral iliac tubercle along with the tensor fasciae latae (TFL) muscle. The fascia lata courses down the lateral aspect of the thigh as two layers, one superficial to and the other deep to the tensor fasciae latae. At the distal end of the TFL, these two layers blend after receiving the insertion of the TFL. This fibrous band continues downward at the iliotibial band and crosses the lateral femoral condyle to split into two elements: the iliopatellar band, and a more distal band that inserts at Gerdy's tubercle on the proximal lateral tibia (see figure 6.29).

The gluteus maximus also inserts into the IT band. According to Ingraham (2018b, para 77),

> Although the gluteus maximus also partially uses the iliotibial band as a tendon, the connection is at an odd angle: the job of the gluteus maximus is probably not to pull directly on the iliotibial band (like most muscle-tendon relationships), but to increase the tension on it by pulling on it laterally (like drawing a bowstring).

Interestingly, some authorities describe the IT band as having a tendinous part that inserts into the lateral femoral condyle, then a ligament that runs from the condyle to Gerdy's tubercle. In this scenario, the IT band is both a long tendon from the TFL and gluteus maximus that attaches to the femur and ligament between the femur and the tibia.

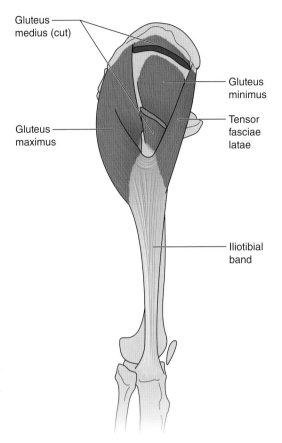

FIGURE 6.29   IT band.

Actions and Function

The IT band functions primarily to stabilize the knee during walking, running, cycling, and so on. As the tendon for the TFL, the IT band assists in abduction, medial rotation, and flexion of the thigh. As the tendon for the gluteus maximus, the IT band may also assist in lateral rotation and extension of the thigh. The IT band also influences patellar tracking through its iliopatellar band and is considered the culprit when the patella tracks too laterally.

Assessment

ROM Testing

Active flexion and extension of the knee, especially against resistance may re-create the athlete's pain as the IT band compresses the fat pad at the femoral condyle. Active abduction of the hip may also be painful.

Manual Resistive Testing

A resisted test for the TFL may cause an increase in the athlete's pain. With the athlete in a side-lying position and the affected hip abducted to approximately shoulder width, the examiner places one hand on the hip and the other just below

FIGURE 6.30   Resisted isometric abduction test.

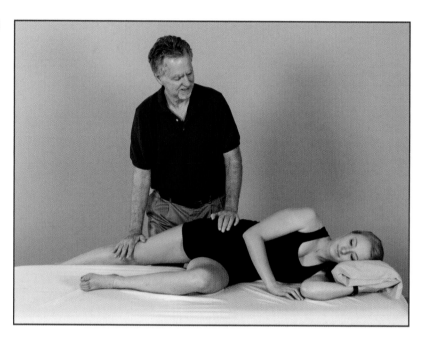

the knee joint (to avoid pressing on the painful tissues) to strongly resist the athlete's attempt to abduct the hip higher (see figure 6.30). This isometric contraction of the TFL and gluteus medius may cause an increase in pain, making this a positive test for IT band syndrome.

Ober's test for tensor fasciae latae hypertonicity and IT band contracture may also be painful if the athlete is experiencing IT band syndrome. Since Dr. Frank Ober first introduced this assessment in 1935, many variations have emerged. One way to perform the test is from a side-lying position on the unaffected side, with the hip and knee flexed to provide stable support and prevent trunk rotation. With the affected hip abducted and slightly extended and the knee flexed to about 20° (this centers the IT band over the trochanter), the examiner stabilizes the pelvis and supports the knee and then directs the athlete to adduct the thigh (this can be passive or active) as if placing the knee behind the other knee (see figure 6.31). A hypertonic TFL or contractured IT band will prevent full adduction. This test may also increase the athlete's pain.

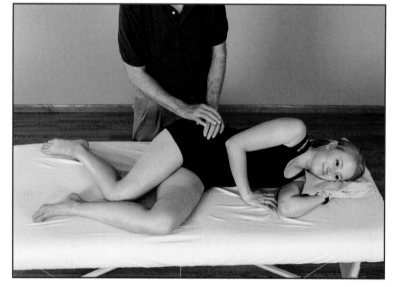

FIGURE 6.31   Ober's test.

Palpatory Examination

Although the athlete can often point to the exact site of pain, palpation is conducted throughout the lateral hip musculature (to identify hypertonicity in the muscle belly) as well as at the distal third of the IT band, including the lateral femoral condyle and Gerdy's tubercle.

Precautions and Contraindications

Rarely, an inflamed synovial pocket is present between the IT band and the superior aspect of the lateral condyle. If massage therapy is administered distal to the knee joint, the practitioner should avoid placing excessive pressure over the common fibular nerve near the fibular head.

Differential Diagnosis

Biceps femoris tendinopathy, lateral collateral ligament sprain, lateral meniscus tear, and superior tibiofibular joint sprain.

Perpetuating Factors

IT band syndrome is caused and perpetuated by many factors, including overtraining and faulty biomechanics. Training factors contributing to this overuse injury may include excessive mileage, sudden increase in training intensity, and poor stretching habits. Biomechanical factors include overpronation, bowlegs, running with the toes pointed in, poor control of knee mechanics, limited ankle ROM, and excessive development of the vastus lateralis, especially in cyclists. Equipment-related factors may include worn outer soles on running shoes, broken-down orthotics, or improper fit on the bike.

Treatment Plan

When ITBS was considered a friction syndrome, the treatment of choice for sports massage therapists was deep transverse friction. Because the evidence overwhelmingly points to ITBS as a compression syndrome, accompanied by weak yet hypertonic tensor fasciae latae and synergistic hip abductor muscles, the treatment has evolved. A typical treatment session is as follows:

1. Administer compressive effleurage and petrissage to the entire lower limb for general warm-up and to reduce the hypertonicity of the surrounding tissues.

2. Administer facilitated stretching of the quadriceps, gluteus maximus, hamstrings, and hip abductor muscles. Combined with the warm-up massage, these stretches help further reduce hypertonicity and the pulling tension on the IT band. At no time are these described as IT band stretches.

3. Because the IT band is a thickened portion of the fascia lata sheath, optimizing the ability of the IT band and underlying tissue to glide on one another promotes the prevention of adhesions that conceivably add to the stresses on the IT band. Specific applications of broad cross-fiber strokes are performed for the quadriceps group, with particular attention to the vastus lateralis underlying the IT band (see figure 6.32). Broad cross-fiber work is also administered to the TFL and gluteus maximus.

4. General anterior–posterior mobilization of the IT band and the underlying vastus lateralis muscle using flat fingers or a loose fist contributes to freer movement between fascial layers (see figure 6.33).

5. Pain-free longitudinal stripping with a loose fist along the IT band (with the intention of accessing the vastus lateralis) may help increase its pliability and improve its ability to glide separately from the vastus lateralis (see figure 6.34).

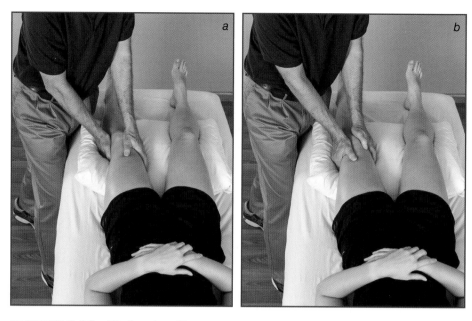

FIGURE 6.32   Bi-directional broad cross-fiber strokes applied to the quadriceps: (a) lateral to medial and (b) medial to lateral.

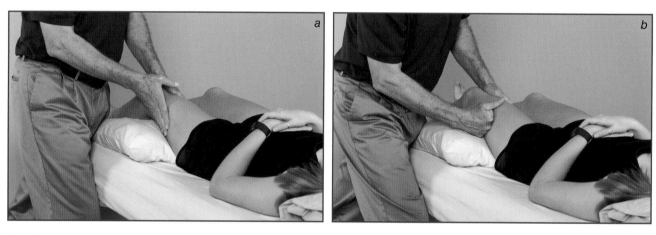

FIGURE 6.33   Mobilizing the IT band in an anterior–posterior direction across the vastus lateralis with (a) flat fingers or (b) a loose fist.

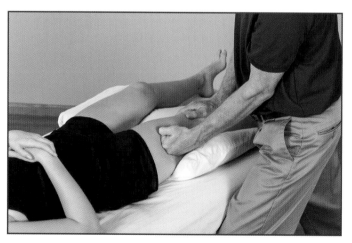

FIGURE 6.34   Loose-fist stripping along the IT band.

6. Apply detailed friction work to the supero-lateral quadriceps tendon (rectus femoris and vastus lateralis) as it merges into the lateral retinaculum (see figure 6.35).

7. Because the section of the IT band from the femoral condyle to Gerdy's tubercle is generally considered to be a ligament, DTF can be applied to the painful areas from the femoral condyle to the insertion on Gerdy's tubercle and to the adjacent lateral retinaculum of the patella (see figure 6.36).

8. Finish the treatment with another round of facilitated stretching for the TFL, gluteus maximus, and synergistic hip abductors.

9. Frequent application of ice is important to help control pain posttreatment.

10. The total number of treatments necessary to resolve the condition depends on the severity of the injury, the frequency of treatment, and the athlete's self-care activities.

FIGURE 6.35   Apply friction to the superolateral quadriceps tendon.

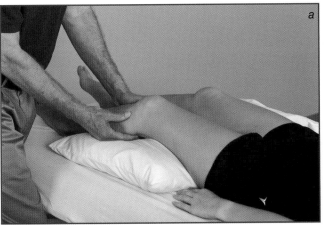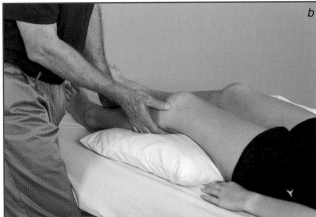

FIGURE 6.36   Apply friction to *(a)* Gerdy's tubercle and *(b)* at the lateral retinaculum.

Self-Care Options

If perpetuating factors are noted, these must be modified or eliminated to reduce the likelihood of recurrence. Because limited flexibility is associated with IT band syndrome, the athlete should consider a self-care program that includes dynamic warm-up before activity and facilitated stretching to improve ROM in hip abduction, hip flexion, hip extension, and internal and external rotation. Attention must also be directed to ankle flexibility because limited dorsiflexion has been correlated to IT band syndrome. Also, because strength imbalances of the hip abductors are associated with IT band syndrome, initiating a program to correct them is crucial to minimizing the risk of another injury.

Case Study

IT Band Syndrome in a Marathon Runner

The client is a 40-year-old female marathon runner who is 2 weeks away from a scheduled marathon. Her complaint is left lateral knee pain with running. She has begun her training taper but expresses concern she will be unable to complete the race. Assessment shows palpatory tightness along left lateral thigh and decreased passive left hip adduction. Treatment consisted of moving massage cupping to the lateral left thigh, followed by broadening strokes to the thigh and cross-fiber strokes to the IT band. Longitudinal stripping was then performed to the tensor fasciae latae and lateral hip musculature.

After release of the targeted tissues, facilitated stretching was performed to the hip abductors and hip flexors, taking the hip into adduction to the point of tissue resistance, then instructing the client to isometrically contract the hip abductors for 10 seconds against the therapist's resistance. On release of the contraction, the hip was adducted to the next point of tissue resistance and the sequence was repeated. Homecare included instruction on self-myofascial release to the TFL and lateral hip musculature with a lacrosse ball or foam roller and self-stretching of hip flexors and abductors. The client was also instructed in hip abductor strengthening exercises to reduce strain on the passive tissues for lateral knee support.

Posttreatment, the client showed increased hip adduction and decreased palpable tension in the lateral thigh. She was able to maintain decreased symptoms through self-care and successfully complete the marathon 2 weeks later.

Earl Wenk, LAT, LMT, ATC, CSCS
Human Performance Collective, LLC, Ann Arbor, Michigan

The medial collateral ligament (MCL) of the knee is one of four major ligaments that stabilize the knee joint. The MCL attaches the medial femoral condyle to the medial tibial condyle and is one of the most commonly injured ligaments of the knee. It's also referred to as the tibial collateral ligament. The main function of the MCL is to resist valgus force on the knee (movement or pressure that gaps the medial femur and the medial tibia).

Signs and Symptoms

The signs and symptoms of an MCL sprain depend on the degree of injury. Generally, the athlete will complain of pain and stiffness on the medial aspect of the knee and may also report instability, as if the knee might give way under stress or the knee might lock or catch. Standing from sitting may reproduce the athlete's pain. Grades 2 and 3 sprains may show signs of swelling, and the athlete might limp. Splinting of the adjacent musculature could help support the medial knee joint. Refer to chapter 4 for detailed descriptions of signs and symptoms of sprains.

Typical History

In collision sports, an acute sprain of the MCL usually occurs as the result of a direct blow to the outside of the knee when the foot is planted, or when the athlete attempts a quick change of direction and the planted foot does not move quickly enough. MCL sprains can also occur when landing from a jump, from a bad fall from a bike, or from simply slipping on a wet or icy road during a run. In more severe sprains, the athlete may report feeling a snap or hearing a tearing sound at the time of injury.

Chronic MCL sprain results from one or more acute sprains that did not heal properly. The chronic condition is usually accompanied by laxity in the MCL. There may also be pain with movements that add a valgus stress to the knee.

Relevant Anatomy

The MCL is a flat band of tough fibrous connective tissue that spans the medial side of the knee from the femoral condyle to the tibial condyle (see figure 6.37). The MCL consists of a deep inner layer that also attaches to the medial meniscus and a superficial band that originates more superior on the medial femoral condyle to an area more inferior on the medial aspect of the tibia. The deep layer of the ligament is prone to becoming injured first and this may lead to a concomitant medial meniscus injury.

Assessment

Observation

The primary indicator of an MCL sprain is the athlete's report of the injury event. The athlete may limp a little or

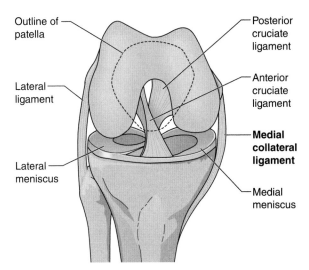

FIGURE 6.37 Medial collateral ligament of the knee.

wince with pain when moving from sitting to standing. Severe sprains may exhibit swelling over the medial knee and into the lower leg.

Manual Resistive Testing

The valgus stress test is used to test for an MCL strain. The athlete is positioned on the examining table with the knee in full extension. The examiner places the cephalad hand against the lateral knee, and the distal hand grasps the ankle. The examiner applies pressure toward the midline to the lateral knee with the cephalad hand while the distal hand pulls the lower leg into abduction (see figure 6.38*a*). This combined motion places a valgus stress on the knee joint, as if gapping the femur and the tibia. The test is repeated with the knee in 30° of flexion (see figure 6.38*b*). Any laxity is compared to the unaffected knee. In the case of an MCL sprain, there will also be tenderness and pain at the medial knee.

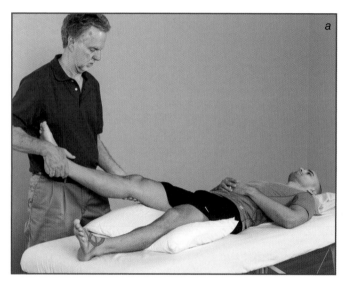
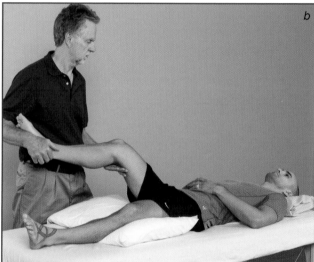

FIGURE 6.38   Valgus stress test: *(a)* straight leg and *(b)* bent knee.

Palpatory Examination

Palpate the ligament and note point tenderness. Typically, the most tenderness is located at the joint line, then the femoral or tibial attachment. The surrounding muscles may be hypertonic and tender, especially at the pes anserine insertions of the gracilis, sartorius, and semitendinosus.

Differential Diagnosis

Medial meniscal tear or injury, anterior cruciate ligament (ACL) tear, tibial plateau fracture, femur injury or fracture, patellar subluxation or dislocation, and medial knee contusion.

Perpetuating Factors

Training factors that contribute to this condition include improper stretching and warm-up, lack of strength training for the hip and knee, and lack of controlled-landing exercises. Biomechanical factors affecting this injury include previous MCL sprains, overpronation, and muscle strength and length issue in the lower extremity and foot.

Treatment Plan

Treatment varies based on whether the injury is acute or chronic.

Treatment of Acute Injury

Acute sprains of any severity can benefit from massage treatment. After physician clearance for grades 2 and 3 sprains and 24 hours after grade 1 sprains, gentle, pain-free effleurage may be administered to help reduce swelling and tenderness around the medial knee. As the swelling and inflammation subside (24–72 hours), the application of gentle, pain-free transverse friction is introduced to stimulate proper scar formation and to prevent adhesions from forming. As healing progresses (swelling and inflammation are gone), transverse friction may be done more firmly but only if pain free. Cyriax (1983) recommends administering transverse friction with the ligament at both ends of its ROM (knee bent and knee straight) to prevent the ligament from forming dysfunctional adhesions to the condyles.

Treatment of Chronic Injury

Once adhesions have formed, deep transverse friction is the method of choice for eliminating them. A typical treatment session for a chronic MCL strain is as follows:

1. Administer compressive effleurage and petrissage and broad cross-fiber strokes to the entire thigh and leg for general warm-up and to reduce the hypertonicity of the medial quadriceps, sartorius, gracilis, and semimembranosus.

2. With the athlete supine, place the knee in pain-free extension and apply DTF to the MCL, paying special attention to the most tender areas. With the knee in extension, the transverse direction is directly anterior–posterior (see figure 6.39a). After 30 to 40 seconds of DTF, place the knee in 30° or more of pain-free flexion and repeat the DTF application. With the knee in flexion, the ligament lies in line with the long axis of the tibia, and the transverse direction is more diagonal (see figure 6.39b).

   The initial application of DTF lasts about 1 minute using moderate pressure, that is, enough pressure to engage the ligament against the

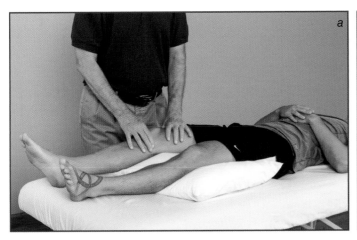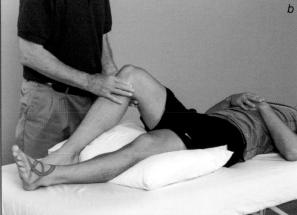

FIGURE 6.39 DTF to the MCL: *(a)* straight leg and *(b)* bent knee.

underlying bone. This may be somewhat painful for the athlete at the beginning, and the practitioner should adjust the pressure to keep the discomfort at about a 6 on a 10-point pain scale. Near the end of the first minute, the discomfort typically will have abated significantly. In some cases, it will remain the same, or it may increase.

3. After the first minute of DTF, the focus shifts to more general massage for the leg muscles addressed in step 1, or perhaps to the uninvolved side, to give time for the treated ligament to rest.

4. Return to the affected area for another round of DTF with the knee in extension and in flexion. This time, the duration of treatment may be up to 3 minutes, as long as the discomfort rating is at or below a 6 on a 10-point scale.

5. Ideally, treatment is given every other day. Following the initial session, the friction portion of subsequent sessions can be longer (up to 9 minutes total) but still given in two or three doses per session. Each dose is given long enough for the pain to subside to near zero.

6. The total duration of treatment depends on the severity of the injury, the frequency of treatment, and the athlete's self-care activities.

Self-Care Options

If perpetuating factors are noted, these must be modified or eliminated to reduce the likelihood of recurrence. Pain-free facilitated stretches for the hamstrings, quadriceps, and adductors help maintain and improve knee extension and flexion. As pain diminishes, a variety of non-weight-bearing strengthening exercises can be added as tolerated. These might include quadriceps setting, straight-leg raises, sitting hip flexion, standing hip extension, standing hamstring curls, and the like. Strength training can then proceed to weight-bearing exercises that focus on stability and resistance to valgus stress.

Patellar tendinopathy, also known as jumper's knee, is an overuse injury associated with running and jumping sports, such as volleyball, basketball, and soccer. Like most overuse injuries, the onset of pain is usually gradual and often ignored until the condition is well advanced.

Signs and Symptoms

Patellar tendinopathy manifests as knee pain localizes to just above or just below the patella. The condition usually develops at the proximal attachment of the tendon on the inferior pole of the patella (see figure 6.40), less commonly at the superior pole, and rarely at the distal attachment on the tibial tubercle. The condition usually presents with little or no swelling. The athlete typically complains of localized pain at the site of the injury and may also report general fatigue in the quadriceps. Pain is typically exacerbated by prolonged weight-bearing knee flexion and by physical activity such as running, playing basketball or volleyball, or participating in modern dance or ballet. The athlete may also report that going up or down stairs causes pain.

Typical History

Patellar tendinopathy is an overuse injury that typically has a gradual onset of pain, appearing from 6 weeks to as long as 3 months after the onset of the offending activity, as degenerative changes develop in the tendon. Athletes with mild to moderate symptoms frequently continue to train and compete, expecting to be able to play through the pain. Athletes who ignore the early signs of tendinopathy and continue to push past the pain will likely contribute to the development of a more severe and problematic condition that will take as long as 3 to 6 months to resolve.

Relevant Anatomy

The patellar tendon attaches the quadriceps muscle group to the tibia via the patella. The portion from the patella to the tibia is also known as the patellar ligament (see figure 6.41).

Assessment

Observation

Visual examination may reveal muscle atrophy of the quadriceps and the gastrocnemius muscles when compared to the unaffected side. According to Rudavsky and Cook (2014, p. 124), "Athletes who continue to train and play, even at an elite level, are not immune to strength and bulk losses, as they are forced to unload because of pain."

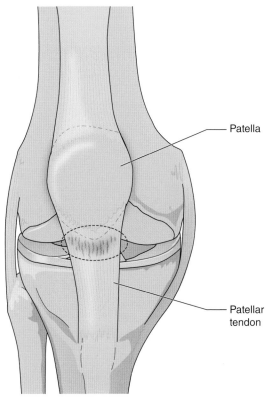

FIGURE 6.40 The inferior pole of the patella is the usual location of tendinopathy.

Patella

Patellar tendon

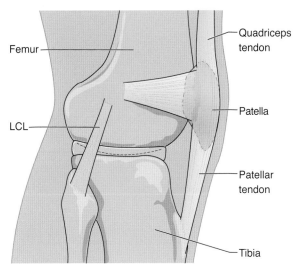

FIGURE 6.41 Patellar tendon.

Femur

LCL

Quadriceps tendon

Patella

Patellar tendon

Tibia

ROM Testing

Reduced flexibility in the hamstrings and quadriceps groups, as well as in ankle dorsiflexion, often accompany (and may be contributory to) patellar tendinopathy.

Manual Resistive Testing

The appropriate muscle test for patellar tendinopathy is resisted knee extension. The athlete can either sit or lie facedown and, beginning with the affected knee flexed to approximately 90°, the examiner resists the athlete's strong isometric contraction of the quadriceps (see figure 6.42). An increase of patellar pain during this test is positive for patellar tendinopathy.

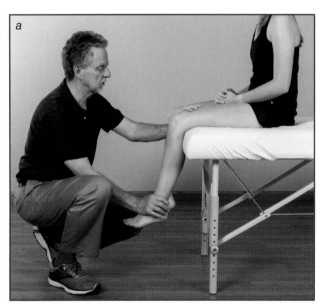
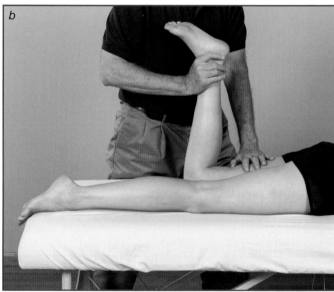

FIGURE 6.42 Resisted knee extension test for patellar tendinopathy: *(a)* sitting and *(b)* lying.

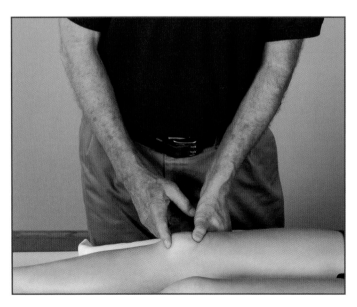

Palpatory Examination

Palpation examination reveals significant, localized pain at the inferior pole of the patella consistent with the pain the athlete is complaining of. Thickening of the tendon may also be noted, but it is rare to see or feel swelling. Accurate palpation is best performed by first anteriorly tilting the inferior pole of the patella and then palpating across the entire inferior edge of the patella (see figure 6.43).

FIGURE 6.43 Palpation of the inferior pole of the tilted patella.

Precautions and Contraindications

Palpation directed posteriorly through the tendon, instead of against the edge of the patella, will engage the infra-patellar bursa (see figure 6.44). Tenderness may also be found here, but indicates bursa irritation, a different condition than the one being assessed.

Differential Diagnosis

Patellofemoral pain syndrome and plica syndrome have many of the same pain characteristics as patellar tendinopathy.

Perpetuating Factors

Training factors may include excessive running mileage, downhill running, repetitive jumping (as in volleyball and basketball), and high-impact aerobics. Biomechanical factors that may contribute to or perpetuate the condition are overpronation, improper tracking of the patella, and rapid strength gains in the quadriceps. Equipment-related factors include worn or broken-down running shoes, poorly fitting orthotics, improper fit on the bike, and aerobic dance on unforgiving floors.

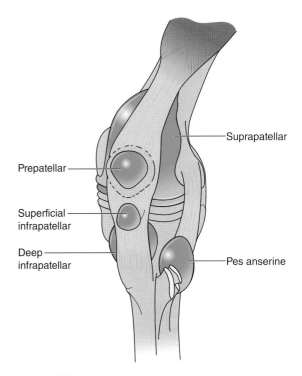

FIGURE 6.44   Infrapatellar bursa.

Treatment Plan

The main component of treatment for this condition is deep transverse friction to the area of the tendon where pain is found on palpation. Friction work is best performed in small doses several times during a session, with two or three sessions per week if possible. A typical treatment session is as follows:

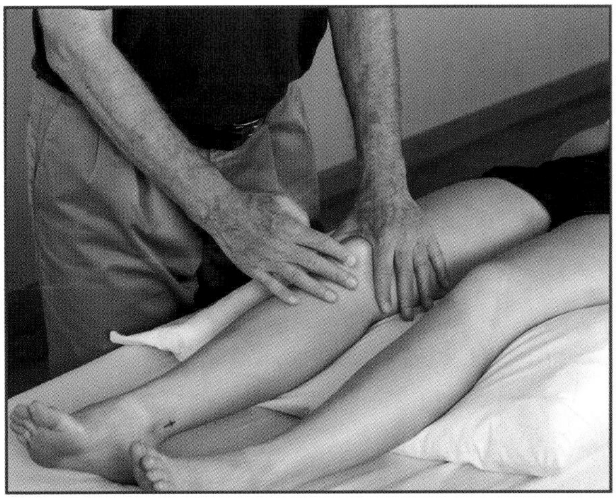

1. Administer compressive effleurage and petrissage to the entire lower limb for general warm-up and to reduce the hypertonicity of the surrounding tissues.

2. Administer facilitated stretching of the quadriceps, hamstrings, and calf muscles. Stretching combined with the warm-up massage helps further reduce hypertonicity and eases the tension on the tendon.

FIGURE 6.45   DTF of the patella.

3. Position the athlete in a comfortable supine position on the treatment table, with only a thin bolster under the knee to allow the knee to fully extend and enable free movement of the patella.

4. To perform DTF effectively, the patella must be properly positioned. Because the most common site for patellar tendinopathy is on the inferior aspect of the patella, tilt the inferior pole anteriorly to access the entire inferior edge of the patella. An easy and comfortable method for doing this is to place the webbing between the thumb and index finger of the nontreating hand against the superior pole and rock the patella posteriorly, that is toward the table (see figure 6.45). This will "pop" the inferior

edge of the patella upward (anteriorly) to allow adequate access to the friction location.

With the inferior pole now accessible, use a braced finger to palpate along the entire edge of the patella. The most painful spot, typically the inferomedial aspect, will be the exact site of the injury and the location to apply DTF to. The initial application of DTF lasts about 1 minute using moderate pressure, that is, enough pressure to engage the tissue and "scrub" it against the bone. This may be somewhat painful for the athlete at the beginning, and the practitioner should adjust the pressure to keep the discomfort at about a 6 on a 10-point pain scale. Near the end of the first minute, the discomfort typically will have abated significantly. In some cases, it will remain the same, or it may increase.

5. At this point, the treatment shifts back to more general massage for the entire lower extremity, or perhaps to the uninvolved side, to give time for the treated tendon to rest.

6. Return to the affected tendon for another round of DTF. This time, the duration of treatment may be up to 3 minutes, as long as the discomfort rating is at or below a 6 on a 10-point scale.

7. Administer pain-free isolytic contractions to help reduce protective inhibition and assist the muscles to return to full activation.

8. Finish the treatment with another round of facilitated stretching for the quadriceps group.

9. Frequent application of ice is important to help control pain posttreatment.

10. Ideally, treatment is given every other day. Following the initial session, the friction portion of subsequent sessions can be longer (up to 9 minutes total) but still given in two or three doses per session. Each dose is given long enough for the pain to subside to near zero.

11. The total duration of treatment depends on the severity of the injury, the frequency of treatment, and the athlete's self-care activities.

Self-Care Options

If perpetuating factors are noted, these must be modified or eliminated to ensure that the injury does not reoccur. Once the tendon pain is eliminated, a program of progressive strengthening can be initiated. A study conducted by Rio and colleagues (2015, p. 1282) found that a single bout of isometric quadriceps exercise reduced patellar tendon pain immediately and for at least 45 minutes afterward. Their findings indicate that "patellar tendon pain affects muscle inhibition and isometric exercise may be used to reduce pain and change muscle inhibition without a reduction in muscle strength." The optimum dosage for an ongoing isometric program has yet to be identified.

A more traditional strengthening program could include non-weight-bearing straight-leg raises, short-arc quadriceps contractions, modified squats (weight-bearing), and other exercises that strengthen the quadriceps muscle–tendon unit and to correct patellar tracking errors. A facilitated-stretching home program for the quadriceps, hip flexors, hamstrings, TFL, and calf muscles is encouraged to help improve ROM and to reduce excessive pull on the patellar tendon.

Triathlete with Knee Pain

An otherwise healthy 54-year-old male presents with right lateral knee and ankle pain. He is not able to run or work out. He is a black belt in Aikido, which he practiced until 10 years ago. He would like to get into triathlons and started training, but the knee pain is debilitating. He also gets many calf cramps through the training. Previously diagnosed with spinal stenosis at C5-C6-C7. He had a car accident 2–3 years ago where he ruptured ligaments in the right medial ankle and injured the right medial knee. Objective examination revealed significant postural and muscle imbalances throughout the lower back, hips, and legs as well as scar tissue over the incision site on the right medial knee.

Treatments consisted of compressive effleurage (evaluating tissue tonicity, hypertonic spots, glide, viscosity), rhythmic compression (increasing blood flow, decreasing overall tonicity), compressive petrissage (increasing fluid presence, separating layers, lifting up tissues), myofascial spreading, and cross-fiber work throughout the musculature of the lower back, hips, legs, and feet. Additionally, specific PNF stretching was incorporated for the hip flexors, hip extensors, and fibularis group. For the knee injury, longitudinal stripping and multidirectional friction was administered to soften the scar tissue and reduce pain.

The athlete's IT band, knee, and hip issues resolved after the initial two months of treatment as he continued training. He started treatment in the beginning of 2015, and the knee pain and IT band issue kept him out of a full Ironman in 2016. He was able to finish a half Ironman in 2016, and a full Ironman in 2017 with a really good time. He has been able to run multiple half marathons and marathons since then with no issues at all. His recovery time was minimal even after longer races. He still comes for post-event massages and maintenance work steadily every 2 weeks in hard training season and once a month off season.

Borbala (Bori) Suranyi, LMT, COMT, CPT
Cape Cod Sports Therapy, Falmouth, MA

Fibularis tendinopathy commonly occurs secondary to an acute or chronic ankle sprain. The muscles involved in this tendinopathy condition are the peroneus longus and the peroneus brevis (also known as the fibularis longus and brevis). The peroneus tertius rarely sustains this injury.

Signs and Symptoms

Tendinopathy may be accompanied by mild swelling and tenderness to the touch at or just proximal to the lateral malleolus. The athlete may report pain or aching that increases with activity such as walking, running, standing on the balls of the feet, and stretching into plantarflexion and inversion. The athlete may report that pain occurs when stretching the muscles by inverting the foot or attempting to evert the foot against resistance.

Typical History

The athlete experiencing fibularis tendinopathy is likely to report a recent lateral ankle sprain or a chronic ankle sprain and instability. As an overuse injury, fibularis tendinopathy develops over a lengthy period, worsening incrementally as the stresses on the tendons continue.

Relevant Anatomy

The fibularis longus arises from the proximal two-thirds of the fibula and courses distally along the fibula, travels posterior to the lateral malleolus, crosses the plantar surface of the foot, and inserts at the base of the first metatarsal and the medial cuneiform on the medial aspect of the longitudinal arch of the foot. The fibularis brevis (deep to the fibularis longus) arises from the distal two-thirds of the fibula and courses posterior to the lateral malleolus to insert at the fifth metatarsal. Together, the fibularis group acts to evert the foot in open-chain activities and to stabilize the foot and ankle in closed-chain activities. They function as "stirrup muscles" in concert with the posterior tibialis to support the longitudinal arch of the foot (see figure 6.46).

The longus and brevis tendons are surrounded by a synovial sheath as they pass behind the lateral malleolus. The sheaths act as a protective sleeve that allows gliding motion of the tendon around the bone, theoretically reducing irritation. Dr. Cyriax and others have theorized that scarring develops on the tendon sheath as a result of acute injury or cumulative microtrauma. This scar tissue then interferes with proper gliding of the tendon, causing irritation and swelling. Cyriax identifies four common sites: one at the myotendinous junction of the fibularis longus and three on the tendon—just proximal, just distal, and at the lateral malleolus (see figure 6.47).

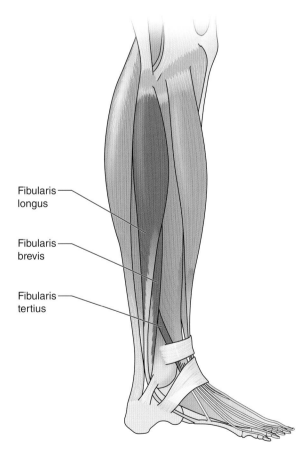

Fibularis longus

Fibularis brevis

Fibularis tertius

FIGURE 6.46 Fibularis group.

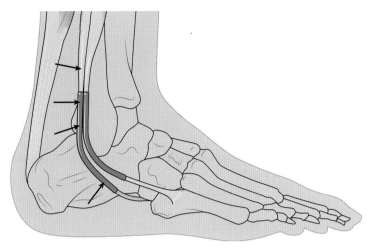

FIGURE 6.47 Typical locations of fibularis tendinopathy.

Assessment

Observation

Visual observation may show mild swelling or redness at the site of the lesion or in the general vicinity. Note the position of the fibularis tendons, which may be visibly malpositioned across or anterior to the malleolus (fibularis subluxation), indicating a torn retinaculum (see figure 6.48).

ROM Testing

Test passive and active plantarflexion, dorsiflexion, inversion, and eversion and note limitations, excessive motion, and pain.

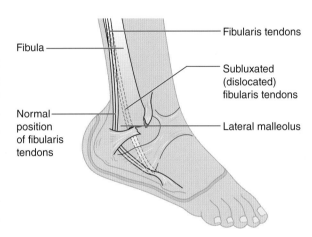

FIGURE 6.48 Subluxed fibularis tendon.

Manual Resistive Testing

Two main isometric muscle tests assess fibularis tendinopathy: resisted eversion with the foot dorsiflexed and resisted eversion with the foot plantarflexed.

The first test, resisted eversion with the foot dorsiflexed, targets the fibularis brevis. Sitting or standing at the foot of the examining table, facing the client's foot, the examiner supports and stabilizes under the heel with the medial hand and places the lateral hand against the lateral aspect of the dorsiflexed foot. The athlete attempts to evert the foot against the examiner's matching resistance (see figure 6.49a). If the fibularis brevis is the affected tissue, the athlete will feel pain at the site of the lesion at the lateral ankle or in the lateral lower leg.

The second test, resisted eversion with the foot plantarflexed, targets the fibularis longus. The examiner maintains the same hand positions as in the previous test, except the foot is fully plantarflexed. The athlete attempts to evert the foot against the examiner's matching resistance (see figure 6.49b). This position isolates the longus more than the brevis. If the fibularis longus is the injured tissue, the athlete will feel pain at the site of the lesion at the lateral ankle or in the lateral lower leg.

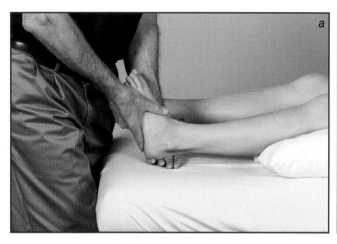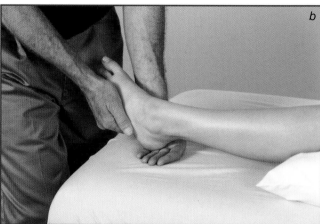

FIGURE 6.49   Resisted eversion test for fibularis tendinopathy: *(a)* the foot in dorsiflexion targets the fibularis brevis and *(b)* the foot in plantarflexion targets the fibularis longus.

Palpatory Examination

The palpatory exam is directed to the area on the tendons that tested positive for pain during the previous aspects of the examination. These are typically located at one or more of the injury sites identified by Cyriax.

Differential Diagnosis

Ankle sprain, ankle impingement syndrome, and ankle fracture.

Perpetuating Factors

Perpetuating factors must be addressed to prevent the recurrence of the injury. If the injury is concurrent with a lateral ankle sprain, full resolution of the sprain is necessary along with rehabilitation of the injured tendons. Working on balance to help retrain the ankle proprioceptors is an important factor to be corrected during recovery. Training factors that contribute to this condition include a sudden increase in exercise intensity or duration, improper stretching and warm-up, and strength imbalances. Biomechanical factors affecting this injury include a rigid, high arch, running and walking on the outside of the feet, and hypertonic fibularis muscles. Equipment-related factors may include worn shoes, shoes with inflexible soles, or shoes with a soft heel counter that fails to stabilize the heel and foot.

Treatment Plan

Deep transverse friction is the primary treatment for fibularis tendinopathy. The severity of the problem and the length of time it's been present are both factors that influence recovery. A typical treatment session is as follows:

1. Administer compressive effleurage and petrissage and broad cross-fiber strokes to the entire lower leg for general warm-up and to reduce the hypertonicity of the fibularis group. Follow with longitudinal stripping to the lateral leg.
2. Pain-free facilitated stretching of the fibularis group helps further reduce hypertonicity and eases the tension on the affected tendon.

3. With the athlete supine, passively invert the foot to place a stretch on the sheathed tendons of the fibularis group. Use the pads of the fingers to administer transverse friction to the tendon or myotendinous junction (see figure 6.50).

The initial application of DTF lasts about 1 minute using moderate pressure. This may be somewhat painful for the athlete at the beginning, and the practitioner should adjust the pressure to keep the discomfort at about a 6 on a 10-point pain scale. Near the end of the first minute, the discomfort typically will have abated significantly. In some cases, it will remain the same, or it may increase.

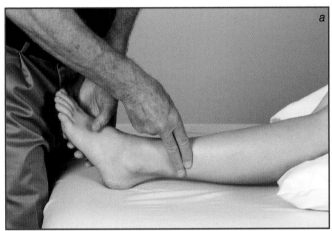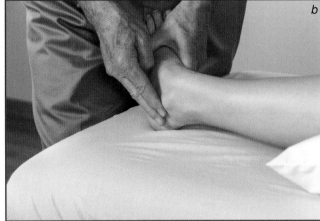

FIGURE 6.50 *(a)* Deep transverse friction to the fibularis longus at the myotendinous junction and *(b)* across the sheathed tendon.

4. After the first minute of DTF, the focus shifts to more general massage for the lower leg, or perhaps to the uninvolved side, to give time for the treated tendon to rest.

5. Return to the affected area for another round of DTF. This time, the duration of treatment may be up to 3 minutes, as long as the discomfort rating is at or below a 6 on a 10-point scale.

6. Administer pain-free isolytic contractions to the fibularis group to help reduce protective inhibition and help the muscles return to full activation.

7. Finish the treatment with another round of facilitated stretching for the fibularis group.

8. Frequent application of ice is important to help control pain posttreatment.

9. Ideally, treatment is given every other day. Following the initial session, the friction portion of subsequent sessions can be longer (up to 9 minutes total) but still given in two or three doses per session. Each dose is given long enough for the pain to subside to near zero.

10. The total duration of treatment depends on the severity of the injury, the frequency of treatment, and the athlete's self-care activities.

Self-Care Options

If perpetuating factors are noted, these must be modified or eliminated to ensure that the injury does not reoccur. Once the tendon pain is eliminated, a program of flexibility and progressive strengthening can be initiated. Swimming, pool running, and easy cycling are good alternative exercises for maintaining fitness while reducing stress on the tendon. When the athlete is pain free, begin strengthening of the fibularis muscles. Start with non-weight-bearing, non-resistive repetitions of eversion from a dorsiflexed position and a plantarflexed position, and then progress to resistive and weight-bearing activities. Stretching should focus on both the fibularis muscles and their antagonists (anterior and posterior tibialis).

Plantar fasciitis is a painful condition of the heel and the plantar aspect of the foot. The classic description of plantar fasciitis assumes that stress on the tissue causes inflammation and mild swelling at its origin on the calcaneus. As with most of the –itis conditions, plantar heel pain has been shown to be a degenerative condition of the collagen that comprises the plantar fascia, and inflammation is typically not present. Therefore, this condition is more appropriately called plantar fasciosis, or fasciopathy (Tahririan et al. 2012; Lemont, Ammirati, and Usen 2003).

Signs and Symptoms

The classic symptom of plantar fascia injury is sharp pain in the heel of the foot during the first few steps after getting out of bed in the morning or after sitting for long periods. The pain tends to diminish with activity, but it may worsen as weight-bearing activities continue. Athletes may also complain of a dull ache in the heel at the end of the day and a feeling of stiffness throughout the foot. Pain is typically felt at the calcaneal attachment, often more medially than centrally. In severe cases, pain may be felt throughout the heel and sole of the foot.

Typical History

This is a condition that has a typical history of onset. Because it can mimic other conditions, such as Baxter's neuropathy, obtaining a detailed history and description of the symptoms is important. Plantar fasciopathy occurs as an overuse injury with the gradual onset of pain at the heel that may radiate into the foot. In many cases of chronic plantar fasciitis, the athlete will have waited months before seeking treatment because the pain "really wasn't too bad" or the pain "goes away as the day goes on" or the pain "hasn't stopped me from training." Athletes may report that a few days or weeks before the onset of their heel pain, they had increased the amount or intensity of athletic activity including running, walking, hiking, and backpacking. Telltale factors include a recent change in shoes, a change in training surface, and other trauma to the foot.

Relevant Anatomy

The plantar fascia (also known as plantar aponeurosis) is a fibrous band of connective tissue (fascia) that arises from the medial calcaneal tubercle and the anterior aspect of the calcaneus and extends along the sole of the foot to attach at the metatarsal arch where it divides into five slips that continue fascially to the toes (see figure 6.51). The plantar fascia is made up of three sections. The central band is the thickest and strongest part, flanked by the smaller and thinner medial and lateral sections. The abductor hallucis muscle has an attachment to the medial band, and the abductor digiti minimi pedis attaches on the lateral band. The flexor digitorum brevis also arises from the calcaneus and is firmly attached to the central band.

The plantar fascia stabilizes the foot and supports the longitudinal arch when weight-bearing. The plantar fascia functions as a spring ligament to dynamically absorb the shock of foot strike and then restore the arch when the foot is unweighted, helping transfer the stored energy during the next step. The plantar fascia is intimately connected

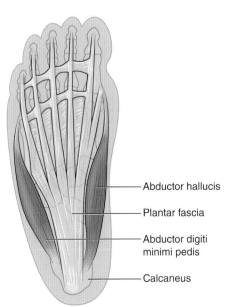

FIGURE 6.51 Plantar fascia.

Abductor hallucis

Plantar fascia

Abductor digiti minimi pedis

Calcaneus

to the calf musculature through the shared fascial plane from the paratenon of the Achilles tendon through the periosteum of the heel (Stecco et al. 2013).

Assessment

ROM Testing

ROM assessment includes active and passive dorsiflexion to check for decreased ROM caused by shortened calf muscles and active and passive toe extension to check for decreased ROM caused by shortened toe flexors. Pain may be reported at the end of range in dorsiflexion and toe extension.

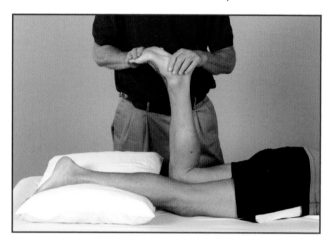

FIGURE 6.52   Resisted toe flexion for plantar fasciopathy.

Manual Resistive Testing

To test for plantar fasciopathy, perform resisted toe flexion. The athlete lies prone on the examining table, with the affected leg flexed at the knee. The examiner supports the foot, passively extends the toes, and then provides graded resistance as the athlete attempts to flex the toes (see figure 6.52). Passive toe extension, especially if combined with dorsiflexion of the foot, may be painful at the end of range.

Palpatory Examination

The palpation exam is conducted throughout the plantar surface of the foot, around the outside edges of the calcaneus (to rule out fat pad syndrome), and around the medial malleolus to determine whether medial tibial nerve entrapment may be present (see figure 6.53). Particular attention is paid to palpation at the calcaneal origin because this is the most common injury area. Thickening of the tissue may also be noted when compared to the unaffected side.

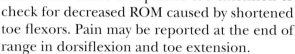
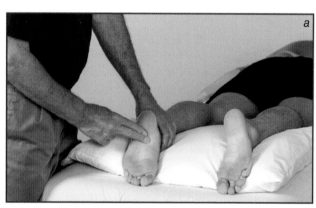
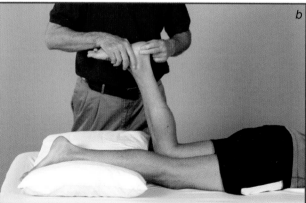
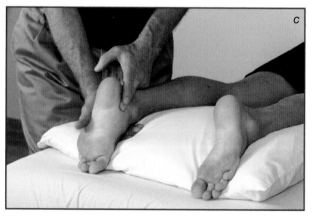

FIGURE 6.53   Palpation of the *(a)* plantar surface of the foot, *(b)* edge of the calcaneus, and *(c)* medial malleolus.

Although not usually palpable, a heel spur may be present at the attachment site. Most authorities agree that a heel spur is more likely a result of plantar fasciitis and not a cause. Occasionally, pain on palpation will be at the anterior aspect of the calcaneus or even in the middle of the central portion. In more severe cases, pain may be reproduced by palpation over the proximal portion of the plantar fascia as it crosses the metatarsal arch. Heel fat pad syndrome, caused by atrophy or loss of elasticity in the fat pad that cushions the calcaneus, may be present (see figure 6.54). If so, palpation may reveal a thinning when compared to the unaffected side and pain to palpation around the borders of the calcaneus. When present, this condition may contribute to the development of plantar fasciitis.

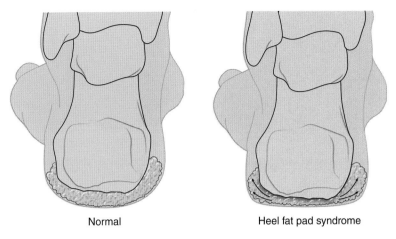

Normal   Heel fat pad syndrome

FIGURE 6.54   Heel fat pad syndrome results in a thinning of the calcaneal fat pad.

Differential Diagnosis

Baxter's neuropathy, bone bruise, calcaneal stress fracture, heel spur syndrome, and heel fat pad syndrome.

Perpetuating Factors

Perpetuating factors must be addressed to prevent the recurrence of the injury. If the condition is the result of excessive pronation of the foot on the affected side, custom orthotics may be necessary. Pelvic imbalance, leg-length discrepancy, and muscle strength and length problems need to be corrected. Training factors that contribute to this condition include sudden increase in training intensity, improper stretching and warm-up, and dancing en pointe. Biomechanical factors affecting this injury include overpronation, a rigid high arch, other biomechanical issues in the foot, and hypertonic calf muscles. Equipment-related factors may include shoes that are worn out, or have too much or too little motion control, shoes with inflexible soles, or shoes with a soft heel counter that fails to stabilize the heel and foot.

Treatment Plan

The severity of the condition and the length of time it's been present are both factors that influence recovery. A typical treatment session is as follows:

1. Administer compressive effleurage and petrissage and broad cross-fiber strokes to the entire lower leg and foot for general warm-up and to reduce the hypertonicity of the calf and foot muscles.
2. Administer facilitated stretching of the calf and the flexors of the foot and toes to further reduce hypertonicity and ease the pulling stress on the plantar fascia.
3. Use braced fingers or thumb to administer deep transverse friction to the most painful area of the plantar fascia as determined in the workup, typically at the origin or just anterior to it (see figure 6.55).

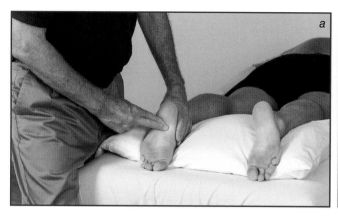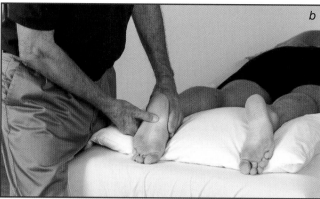

FIGURE 6.55   DTF of plantar fascia: *(a)* braced finger and *(b)* thumb.

The initial application of DTF lasts about 1 minute using moderate pressure, that is, enough pressure to "scrub" the tissue against the underlying bone. This may be somewhat painful for the athlete at the beginning, and the practitioner should adjust the pressure to keep the discomfort at about a 6 on a 10-point pain scale. Near the end of the first minute, the discomfort typically will have abated significantly. In some cases, it will remain the same, or it may increase.

4. After the first minute of DTF, the focus shifts to more general massage for the foot, or perhaps to the uninvolved side, to give time for the treated tissues to rest.

5. Return to the affected area for another round of DTF. This time, the duration of treatment may be up to 3 minutes, as long as the discomfort rating is at or below a 6 on a 10-point scale.

6. Administer pain-free pin-and-stretch work to the plantarflexors of the foot and toes.

7. Finish the treatment with another round of facilitated stretching for the calf muscles.

8. Frequent application of ice is important to help control pain posttreatment.

9. Ideally, treatment is given every other day. Following the initial session, the friction portion of subsequent sessions can be longer (up to 9 minutes total) but still given in two or three doses per session. Each dose is given long enough for the pain to subside to near zero.

10. The total duration of treatment depends on the severity of the injury, the frequency of treatment, and the athlete's self-care activities.

Self-Care Options

If perpetuating factors are noted, these must be modified or eliminated to ensure that the injury does not reoccur. Specially designed night splints to maintain a mild stretch on the plantar tissues of the foot have proven effective in some cases. Self-administered massage combined with cryotherapy is performed by freezing water in a 16 oz. (.5 l) plastic bottle and rolling the bottom of the foot (see figure 6.56). As healing progresses, the ice-bottle can be supplanted by a tennis ball, golf ball, or one of a variety of foot rollers commercially available.

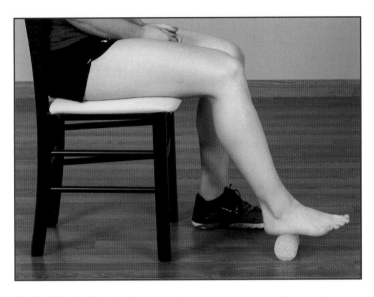

FIGURE 6.56 Self-administered massage with cryotherapy using a frozen bottle of water.

Once the heel pain is eliminated, initiate a program of flexibility and progressive strengthening. Stretching exercises should focus on foot mobility and improving dorsiflexion. Easy strengthening exercises for the foot include picking up marbles with the toes (see figure 6.57a), using the toes to scrunch a small towel under the foot (see figure 6.57b), and walking barefoot in sand. Swimming, pool running, and easy cycling are good alternative exercises for maintaining fitness while reducing stress on the plantar fascia. The athlete should not run again until calf raises are pain free.

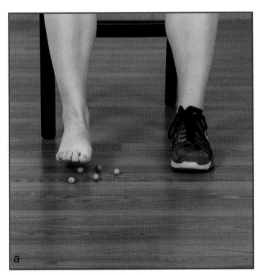
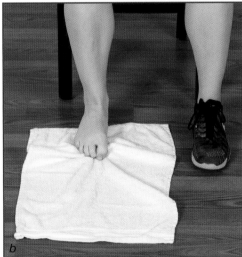

FIGURE 6.57 Strengthening exercises for the foot: *(a)* marble pick-up and *(b)* towel scrunch.

Marathon Runner With Ruptured Plantar Fascia

The client is a 24-year-old elite female runner who ruptured her right plantar fascia 6 months ago and has not been able to run. She rates her pain as 8 to 9 on the pain scale and reports dull, knifelike pain and throbbing. She presents with pain in the arch of the right foot, traveling from the heel of the foot along the medial aspect of the foot and up to the ankle and lower leg. She has had many years of sporadic plantar pain and dealt with it with stretching, massage, and rest. She has been using ice–heat contrast therapy, foot rolling, and massage for pain control. When she wakes up in the morning, it's stiff and painful to walk. When she warms up the soft tissues with either rolling out the plantar surface of her foot with a ball, massage, heat, and slow walking, it feels better.

She has decreased range of motion. Dorsiflexion in particular was severely limited compared to the contralateral ankle. Passive range of motion does not cause pain; however, pain is elicited with active range of motion. The flexor hallucis longus and brevis are severely hypertonic and thickened. Treatment consists of 15- to 30-minute sessions performed at least four times weekly for 6 weeks.

The tissue was warmed with effleurage, and then direct digital pressure was applied on the insertion of the flexor hallucis brevis with digital pressure pin and stretch and active engagement of the antagonist muscles in the anterior compartment of the lower leg. Additionally, effleurage and petrissage of the superficial and deep flexor and posterior muscles were administered, giving special attention to the tendons of the flexors around the ankles. Lastly, pin and stretch and active engagement of specific sites were performed.

Self-massage with lacrosse balls, golf balls, and foam rollers in combination with electronic stimulation and cold compression was used to complement the treatment after exercise and throughout the day.

Over the course of this intensive 6-week therapeutic intervention, this athlete was able to return to elite running at top performance, breaking marathon records. She continues receiving regular bodywork sessions. She has maintained her home program of self-massage, electronic stimulation and cold compression, and exercises using resistance bands to maintain overall foot and ankle strength and stability.

Michael Moore, CMT, BCTMB, ART® Provider
Integrative Bodywork Institute, Shell Beach, California

Shin splints is a catch-all term for lower-leg pain with no other obvious etiology. When the injury is on the medial side of the shin, it's usually attributed to stress in the posterior tibialis muscle and tendons, and the medical diagnosis is medial tibial stress syndrome or MTSS. Pain on the lateral tibia may also be categorized and diagnosed as shin splints. Lateral tibia pain is usually attributed to stress in the muscle belly or the tibial attachments of the anterior tibialis. This injury affects many types of athletes, including runners, tennis players, dancers, high-impact aerobics participants, and military recruits.

Signs and Symptoms

Shin splints are reported as a dull ache, tenderness, soreness, or pain along the tibia, either medially or laterally (see figure 6.58). Pain may also be accompanied by mild swelling in the lower leg. The most common site for shin splints is along the distal aspect of the medial tibia.

Typical History

As in most overuse injuries, the onset of shin splints pain is gradual. There may be pain at the start of exercise activity, which often eases as the tissues warm up, then comes back near the end of the training session or afterward. Shin splints often occur in beginning runners who do too many miles too soon or in experienced runners who abruptly change their workout, for example increasing mileage by more than 10% per week, or switching from running on flat surfaces to running on hills. Military recruits often experience shin splints during basic training because of the intensity of training combined with inadequate footwear.

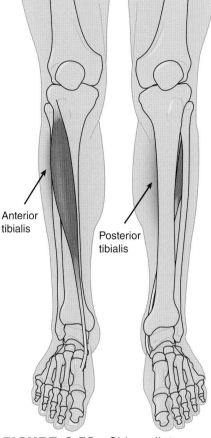

FIGURE 6.58 Shin splints can occur at the medial or lateral tibia.

Anterior tibialis

Posterior tibialis

Relevant Anatomy

The primary muscles involved in shin splints are the tibialis anterior and posterior. The tibialis anterior arises from the lateral tibial condyle and the proximal two-thirds of the shaft of the tibia and its interosseous membrane and inserts at the base of the first metatarsal and the first cuneiform (see figure 6.59a). The tibialis posterior is located in the deep posterior compartment and is the deepest muscle in the calf. It arises from the proximal two-thirds of the posterolateral tibia, posteromedial fibula, and interosseous membrane (see figure 6.59b). It inserts on the medial plantar foot (navicular; medial cuneiform; cuboid, calcaneus; and second, third, and fourth metatarsals).

Actions and Function

When the foot is free to move, the tibialis anterior dorsiflexes and inverts it. When the foot is on the ground (closed-chain activities), the tibialis anterior assists in maintaining balance. During walking or running, tibialis anterior lifts the foot to clear the ground as the leg swings forward and helps prevent the foot from slapping onto the ground after heel strike (eccentric activation). When the foot is free to move, the tibialis posterior inverts it and assists plantarflexion.

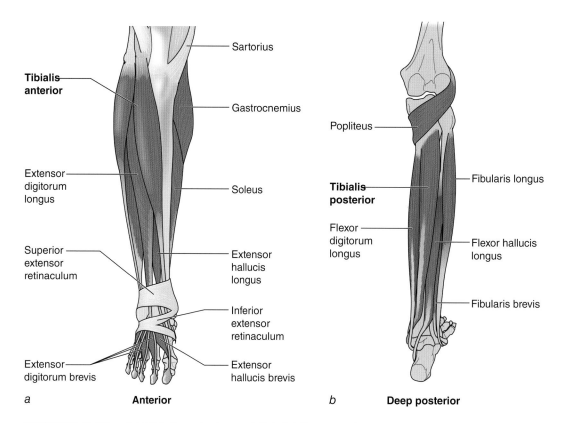

FIGURE 6.59   *(a)* Tibialis anterior and *(b)* tibialis posterior.

When the foot is on the ground (closed-chain activities), the tibialis posterior assists in maintaining balance and stabilizing the medial longitudinal arch, helping to control pronation.

Assessment

ROM Testing

Range may be limited because of pain, either with an active contraction or during a passive stretch of the affected tissues. The tibialis anterior's normal ROM for plantarflexion (lengthening direction) is 50° and for dorsiflexion (shortening direction) is 20°. The tibialis posterior's normal ROM for inversion (shortening direction) is 45° and for eversion (lengthening direction) is 20°.

Manual Resistive Testing

The appropriate muscle test for shin splints depends on the location of the pain because the source can be either the anterior or posterior tibialis. To test the tibialis anterior, the foot of the affected leg is dorsiflexed approximately 90° (relative neutral), and the examiner resists the athlete's strong isometric contraction of the anterior tibialis (dorsiflexion and inversion) (see figure 6.60*a*). If the complaint is caused by the anterior tibialis, an increase in pain will most likely be noted at the myotendinous junction or in the muscle belly along the lateral tibia.

To test the tibialis posterior, the foot of the affected leg is dorsiflexed approximately 90° (relative neutral), and the examiner resists the athlete's strong isometric contraction of the posterior tibialis (inversion only) (see figure 6.60*b*). If the complaint is caused by the posterior tibialis, an increase in pain will most likely be noted at the myotendinous junction or in the distal muscle belly along the medial tibia.

Palpatory Examination

The palpation exam is guided by the findings from the patient history, the ROM assessments, and the muscle testing. Pain present on palpation indicates an active injury process. The examiner assesses the pain the athlete is complaining of and then determines the most painful area within that region.

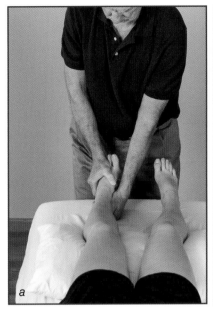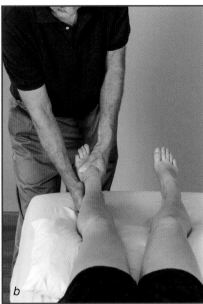

FIGURE 6.60 *(a)* Resisted dorsiflexion and inversion tests tibialis anterior and *(b)* resisted inversion tests tibialis posterior.

Differential Diagnosis

Compartment syndrome and tibial stress fracture.

Perpetuating Factors

Training factors include running and jumping activities (such as high-impact aerobics), especially on cement floors and with inadequate foot support (worn shoes, dancing barefoot), which may contribute to and perpetuate the development of shin splints. Runners who run on banked tracks or always run on the same side of a cambered road may also develop this injury. This condition may also manifest as a result of uphill running. Biomechanical factors such as flat feet or weak arches, both of which cause undue stretch on the muscles and tendons of the lower-leg muscles, will perpetuate shin splints. Weakness in the anterior or posterior tibialis will also contribute to this injury. Equipment-related factors include worn or broken-down running shoes or poorly fitting orthotics.

Treatment Plan

Shin splints caused by anterior tibialis overuse can be successfully treated using deep transverse friction to the area of the muscle and tendon where pain is revealed through palpation. Friction work is best performed in small doses several times during a session, with two or three sessions per week if possible. When treated this way, even long-standing tendinopathy responds favorably in a relatively short time. A typical treatment session is as follows:

1. Administer compressive effleurage and petrissage to the entire lower limb for general warm-up and to reduce the hypertonicity of the surrounding tissues.

2. Administer facilitated stretching of the muscle groups of the lower leg and ankle. Stretching combined with the warm-up massage helps further reduce hypertonicity and eases the tension on the tendons.

3. To treat the tibialis anterior if the lesion is in the muscle belly (rarely) or at the distal myotendinous junction (frequently), administer focused compressive petrissage and broad cross-fiber strokes to the muscle belly before friction. Administering pin and stretch to the muscle belly may also be useful. Transverse friction is effectively delivered by standing opposite the affected leg, stabilizing with one hand at the neutral ankle, and using the flats of the fingers of the other hand to administer the stroke (see figure 6.61). To spare the finger joints, hold the fingers stiffly and move the arm to produce the sweep of the stroke.

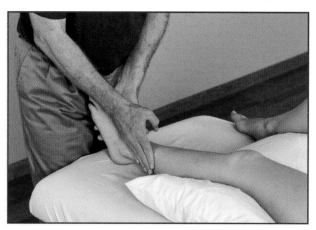

FIGURE 6.61   DTF of the tibialis anterior myotendinous junction.

The initial application of DTF lasts about 1 minute using moderate pressure, that is, enough pressure to engage the tissue and "scrub" it against the bone. This may be somewhat painful for the athlete at the beginning, and the practitioner should adjust the pressure to keep the discomfort at about a 6 on a 10-point pain scale. Near the end of the first minute, the discomfort typically will have abated significantly. In some cases, it will remain the same, or it may increase.

4. Shin splints caused by tibialis posterior overuse are difficult to treat because the muscle belly is deep behind the tibia. Compressive petrissage and broad cross-fiber strokes along the medial tibia will help increase circulation and relax the muscles adjacent to the posterior tibialis. Longitudinal stripping strokes along the medial aspect of the tibia seem to worsen the condition.

The tendon of the tibialis posterior is palpable as it emerges from behind the tibia several inches (5 cm) proximal to the medial malleolus. This is a sheathed tendon and subject to tenosynovitis. According to Cyriax (1983, 18), in tenosynovitis "the sheath becomes roughened and inflamed from overuse." For this reason, the tendon is treated on a stretch, to provide a firm surface to rub the sheath against as a way to smooth its roughened and irritated surfaces.

Deep transverse friction is administered to the sheathed tendon by grasping the foot with the nontreating hand and everting the foot to stretch the tendon. Palpation with the treating hand reveals the exact site of the lesion (there may be more than one). Friction is performed by using the flats of the fingers to apply moderate pressure against the tendon and then moving in a cross-fiber direction to treat the lesion (see figure 6.62).

5. After the first minute of DTF, the focus shifts to more general massage for the entire lower extremity, or perhaps to the uninvolved side, to give time for the treated tissues to rest.

6. Return to the affected area for another round of DTF. This time, the duration of treatment may be up to 3 minutes, as long as the discomfort rating is at or below a 6 on a 10-point scale.

7. Administer pain-free isolytic contractions to help reduce protective inhibition and help the muscles return to full activation.

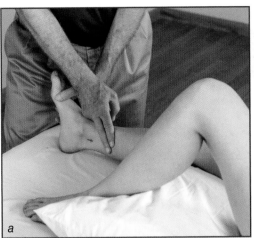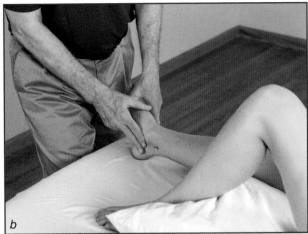

FIGURE 6.62   DTF of the tibialis posterior at *(a)* the myotendinous junction and at *(b)* the medial malleolus.

8. Finish the treatment with another round of facilitated stretching for the hamstrings and calf muscles.

9. Frequent application of ice is important to help control pain posttreatment.

10. Ideally, treatment is given every other day. Following the initial session, the friction portion of subsequent sessions can be longer (up to 9 minutes total) but still given in two or three doses per session. Each dose is given long enough for the pain to subside to near zero.

11. The total duration of treatment depends on the severity of the injury, the frequency of treatment, and the athlete's self-care activities.

Self-Care Options

If perpetuating factors are noted, these must be modified or eliminated to ensure that the injury does not reoccur. Once the pain is eliminated, initiate a program of flexibility and progressive strengthening.

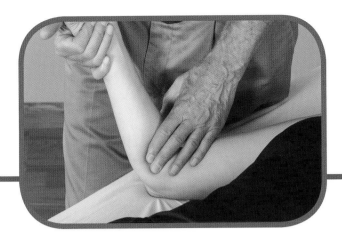

Chapter 7

Treatment of Upper-Extremity Soft Tissue Injuries

Upper-extremity soft tissue injuries affect many athletes involved in throwing and racket sports, swimming, and gymnastics. These complaints are also common in nonathletes whose work or leisure activities place heavy stress on the shoulder girdle and arms. This chapter discusses four common overuse injuries and offers a sports massage approach to treating them. Please note that many possible treatment scenarios are appropriate for the injuries presented here. The suggested treatment progressions for each injury discussed in this chapter are the author's preferred approaches.

The rotator cuff is made up of the tendons of four muscles: subscapularis, supraspinatus, infraspinatus, and teres minor (see figure 7.1). In concert with the ligaments around the shoulder joint, the rotator cuff helps to stabilize the humeral head in the glenoid fossa. These four muscles, acting synergistically with other dynamic stabilizers that attach to the scapula and humerus, also act to efficiently move the humerus through its ranges of motion.

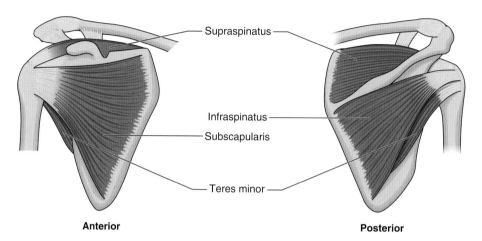

Anterior   **Posterior**

FIGURE 7.1 Rotator cuff.

Injuries to the rotator cuff most commonly occur as tendinopathy, impingement syndromes, or tears. The supraspinatus is the most commonly injured of the rotator cuff group. The focus of discussion in this section is on tendinopathy of the rotator cuff. Tendinopathy is typically an overuse injury that develops over months before overt symptoms appear. Usually, these symptoms appear gradually; sometimes they flare up suddenly, especially as a result of increased intensity in training or a change in training.

Signs and Symptoms

Because this is an overuse injury, the pain of rotator cuff tendinopathy comes on gradually, generally with the feeling of a deep ache in the affected shoulder and becomes worse over time, aggravated by lifting the arm into abduction or putting the arm behind the back (internal rotation). The athlete may also report pain during sleep, particularly if lying on the affected shoulder. Painful clicking or crepitus may occur with movement.

Typical History

Tears of the rotator cuff are sometimes traumatic. The client will be able to pinpoint the moment the injury occurred. More commonly, tears develop as a result of repetitive, eccentric overload. An eccentric contraction occurs when the muscle contracts as it resists being lengthened. This is sometimes called *negative work*. It also occurs as muscles decelerate motion, as in throwing, racket sports, downhill running, and kicking.

Impingement syndromes and tendinopathy are more insidious, although they can suddenly flare up as a result of increased intensity or duration of the causative activity. Tendinopathy may also be accompanied by subacromial bursitis, which complicates the assessment and treatment. Referred pain at the shoulder is also quite common and can lead to confusing or inconclusive assessment test results.

Relevant Anatomy

Subscapularis

The subscapularis originates on the anterior scapula, filling the subscapular fossa and inserts into the lesser tubercle of the anterior humerus. Actions include internal (medial) rotation of the humerus, assisting adduction of the humerus, and assisting stabilization of the humeral head in the glenoid fossa during other motions of the humerus.

Supraspinatus

The supraspinatus originates in the supraspinous fossa of the scapula and inserts into the superior aspect of the greater tubercle of the humerus. Actions include abduction of the humerus and stabilization of the humeral head in the glenoid fossa when the arm is hanging at the side, especially if weighted.

Infraspinatus

The infraspinatus originates on the infraspinous fossa of the scapula and inserts into the posterior aspect of the greater tubercle of the humerus. Actions include lateral (external) rotation of the humerus, assisting in abduction of the humerus, and stabilization of the head of the humerus in the glenoid fossa during upward movement.

Teres Minor

The teres minor originates on the posterior, lateral scapula and inserts into the posterior aspect of the greater tubercle of the humerus, inferior to and blended with the infraspinatus tendon. The teres minor is separated from the teres major by the tendon of the long head of the triceps as it passes to its attachment on the infraglenoid tubercle. Actions include lateral (external) rotation of the humerus, assisting abduction of the humerus, and stabilization of the head of the humerus in the glenoid fossa during upward movement.

Assessment

Injuries at the shoulder can be extremely difficult to pinpoint. Because shoulder pain can be referred from structures in the neck as well as trigger points in the cervical and upper-back muscles, in addition to pain that's actually coming from an injury to the shoulder, these assessments may or may not isolate the problem definitively.

Observation

With the client standing relaxed, look for imbalances in shoulder elevation, anterior and posterior deviation, and medial rotation. In chronic cases, atrophy of the deltoid muscles may be noticeable. With the arms hanging at the sides, the

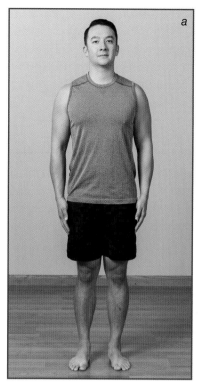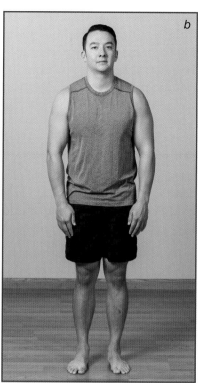

FIGURE 7.2 *(a)* When shoulders are relaxed, thumbs face forward, indicating the arms in neutral. *(b)* Excessive medial rotation of the humerus will cause the backs of the hands to face forward.

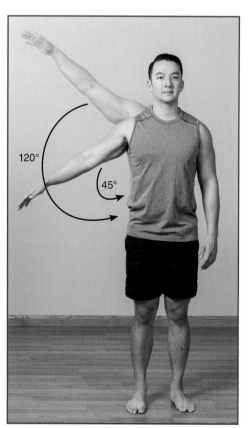

thumbs should face forward (see figure 7.2*a*). If there is excessive medial rotation, the backs of the hands will face forward (see figure 7.2*b*). Exercises with the humerus in medial rotation (like the butterfly stroke in swimming and upright rows in weight training) are the most frequent cause of impingement syndromes.

ROM Assessment

Active ROM movements at the shoulder consist of flexion, extension, abduction, adduction, horizontal abduction, and horizontal adduction. During active ROM, look for altered motion as a reaction to pain. Passive motion is generally pain free, although in more severe cases of rotator cuff tendinopathy, the tendon structures may be pinched under the acromion as the humerus moves. Resisted tests should produce pain when the muscle tendon unit at fault is tested.

During ROM testing, both active and passive, the athlete may experience pain between 45° and 120° of abduction. This painful arc may be the result of subacromial bursitis, bone spurs, or tendinopathy in the rotator cuff (see figure 7.3). The pain is caused

FIGURE 7.3 A painful arc may be present between about 45° and 120° of abduction.

by the pinching of injured tissues under the acromion process or the coracoacromial ligament or both. When a painful arc is present and resisted tests performed with the joint in neutral are negative, the pain is likely caused by bursitis. When a painful arc is present and resisted tests are positive, the pain is likely caused by contractile tissue being pinched during movement.

Manual Resistive Tests

Supraspinatus

The athlete stands comfortably, with her arms hanging at her sides. The examiner presses the arm to be tested against the athlete, while stabilizing her on the opposite hip. The athlete begins slowly to try to abduct the arm, continuing to build to a strong isometric contraction of the supraspinatus against the examiner's resistance (see figure 7.4). Pain or weakness is considered a positive test.

It's also recommended to perform the "empty can" test for supraspinatus involvement. In this test, the athlete raises both arms into about 90° abduction and 30° forward flexion (in the scapular plane), with the thumbs pointed toward the floor (humeral internal rotation) as if pouring out a beverage container (empty can). The examiner presses downward against the forearms while the athlete resists (see figure 7.5). Pain or weakness is a positive result for supraspinatus injury. In some cases, there is no pain during the isometric resistance, but there is pain on the release. This is considered to be a positive test.

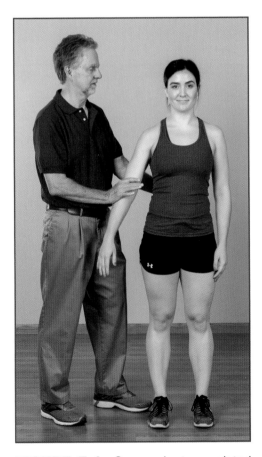

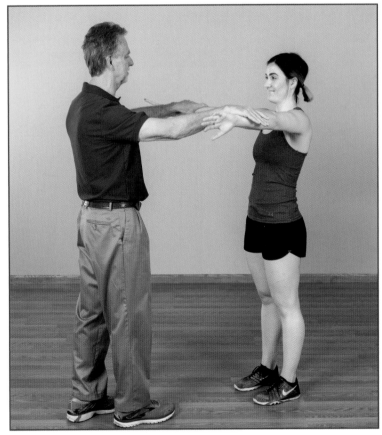

FIGURE 7.4 Supraspinatus resisted test.

FIGURE 7.5 Empty can test for supraspinatus.

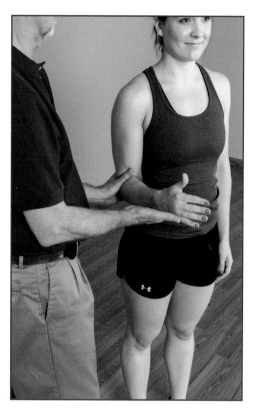

FIGURE 7.6 Subscapularis resisted test.

Subscapularis

This test is best performed with the athlete standing, holding the arm of the affected shoulder against her side and flexing the elbow to 90°. The examiner stabilizes the humerus against the athlete so they cannot abduct their arm. With the other hand, the examiner grasps across the medial wrist to provide resistance to the athlete's isometric internal rotation (see figure 7.6). The athlete begins slowly to try to pull her wrist toward her abdomen, as if swinging her arm inward like a gate, continuing to build to a strong isometric contraction of the subscapularis. Pain or weakness is considered a positive test. If pain does not increase during the first test position, repeat the test again with the subscapularis on more of a stretch by rotating the humerus externally to 135° and retesting, then to 180° and retesting. Each position progressively increases the stress on the muscle–tendon unit.

It's also recommended to perform Gerber's lift-off test to assess the subscapularis. In this test, the athlete positions the arm behind the back, with the palm facing out. The examiner directs the athlete to lift the hand off the back, increasing internal rotation of the humerus (see figure 7.7*a*). In some versions of this test, the examiner pushes against the hand to increase the activation of the subscapularis (see figure 7.7*b*). Pain or weakness is considered positive for subscapularis injury.

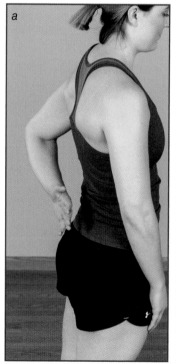
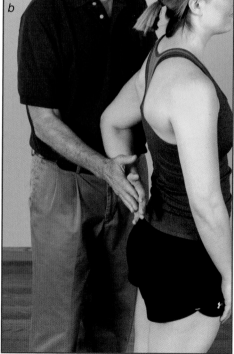

FIGURE 7.7 Gerber's lift-off test.

Infraspinatus and Teres Minor

This test starts in the same position as the subscapularis test, with the athlete standing, holding the arm of the affected shoulder against her side and flexing the elbow to 90°. The examiner stabilizes the humerus against the athlete so she cannot abduct her arm. With the other hand, the examiner grasps across the lateral wrist to provide resistance to the athlete's isometric external rotation (see figure 7.8a). Because the infraspinatus and teres minor are external rotators of the humerus, the athlete attempts to externally rotate against the examiner's resistance. Care must be taken to ensure that she is swinging her arm like a gate, not trying to abduct the arm. If no increase in pain is felt during the first test position, repeat the test again with the muscles on more of a stretch. Rotate the humerus

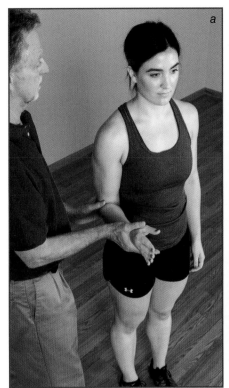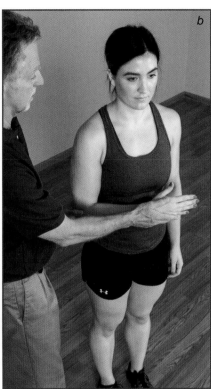

FIGURE 7.8 Infraspinatus and teres minor resisted test, performed in (a) a neutral position and (b) humerus internally rotated.

internally to 45° and retest, then to 20° and retest (see figure 7.8b). Each position progressively increases the stress on the infraspinatus and teres minor muscle–tendon units.

Palpation

Because of the prevalence of referred pain at the shoulder, palpation is of little value before functional testing, which is designed to isolate the structures that are the source of the pain. Once the tissue at fault is determined, palpation can be limited to that tissue. The examiner can then be guided by the athlete's report of pain or tenderness during palpation for the causative lesion, which is usually the most tender spot.

Supraspinatus

The supraspinatus tendon lies under the acromion process. The athlete must be positioned so that she can comfortably medially rotate, adduct, and hyperextend the humerus (hammerlock position with the forearm held away from the back) to expose the tendon. This can be done from a sitting or side-lying position. The tendon is palpated lateral and parallel to the bicipital groove and just inferior to the anterolateral border of the acromion. Light transverse friction is administered horizontally across the now almost vertical tendon.

To access the myotendinous junction of the supraspinatus, the athlete's arm is supported in 90° of abduction if this can be accomplished without pain. In this position, the myotendinous junction lies directly deep to the V formed by the clavicle and spine of the scapula. Now that the upper trapezius is relaxed, palpation through it to the supraspinatus is possible (see figure 7.9). Light friction is accomplished with a braced finger using a rolling motion by pronating and supinating the forearm.

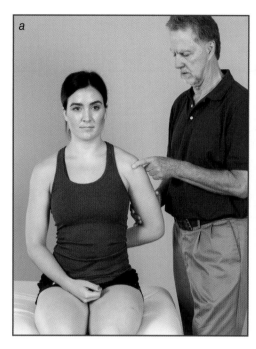
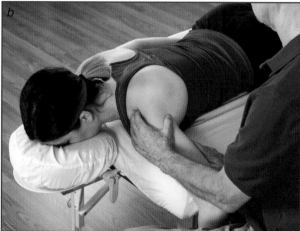

FIGURE 7.9 *(a)* Palpation of the supraspinatus tendon attachment and *(b)* the MT junction.

Subscapularis

The athlete lies supine, with the hand of the affected arm resting on the thigh. This position places the bicipital groove of the humerus directly anterior, that is, facing the ceiling.

With the arm in this position, the examiner palpates to locate the coracoid process, then moves laterally and inferiorly toward the head of the humerus (see figure 7.10). The subscapularis tendon attaches at the lesser tuberosity, just medial to the bicipital groove. The tendon is partially covered medially by the tendons of the coracobrachialis and the short head of the biceps and laterally by the edge of the anterior deltoid. Care must be taken to move these structures out of the way to directly contact the subscapularis tendon. Light transverse friction is administered in a superior–inferior direction because the tendon attaches horizontally. Once located, more of the tendon can be accessed by rotating the humerus a few degrees laterally.

Infraspinatus and Teres Minor

The infraspinatus and teres minor blended tendon may be partially covered by the spine of the scapula at the acromion. The athlete must be positioned to comfortably move the tendon from under the acromion to make it accessible to palpation. The best positioning has the athlete sitting or prone on elbows with the shoulder in 90° flexion, 10° adduction, and 20° lateral rotation. The infraspinatus tendon is palpated just inferior to the posterolateral corner of the acromion (see figure 7.11). Another option has the athlete prone on the treatment table, with their

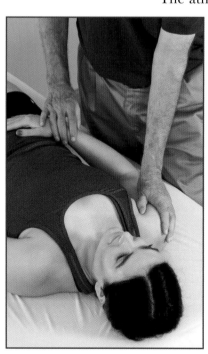

FIGURE 7.10 Palpation of the subscapularis tendon.

face resting in the face cradle. The affected arm hangs over the front edge of the table in adduction and lateral rotation. In either position, it is now possible to palpate the tendon on the posterior humerus, seeking the most tender area. Light transverse friction is administered perpendicular to the shaft of the humerus. The teres minor attaches just inferior to and blends with the infraspinatus. Although it is rarely at fault, friction may be administered to it to palpate for tenderness.

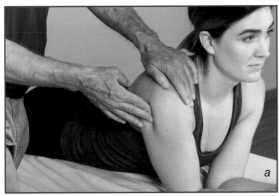
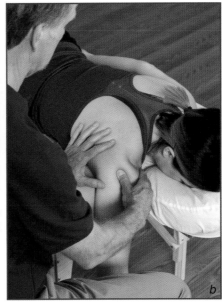

FIGURE 7.11 Palpation of the infraspinatus tendon *(a)* with athlete supported on elbows and *(b)* prone on the treatment table.

Precautions and Contraindications

Subacromial bursitis can be exacerbated by massage.

Differential Diagnosis

Calcific tendinopathy, subacromial bursitis, biceps brachii tendinopathy, acromioclavicular joint injury, and cervical radiculopathy.

Perpetuating Factors

Tendinopathy at the rotator cuff can be accompanied by bursitis, which muddies the assessment process and complicates the treatment. The bursitis may not become apparent until the tendinopathy is well on its way to being resolved and vice versa. Impingement syndrome, in which soft tissue structures are pinched as they pass under the acromion or the ligamentous acromial arch, can also interfere with proper healing. Muscular imbalance, especially between the medial and lateral rotators, must be addressed if proper healing is to occur and to help prevent recurrence of the injury.

Treatment Plan

Deep transverse friction is the primary treatment for rotator cuff tendinopathy and can be sandwiched between preparatory strokes and finishing techniques. The severity of the condition and the length of time it has been present are both factors that influence recovery.

A typical treatment session is as follows:

1. Apply compressive effleurage and petrissage and broad cross-fiber work to the upper extremity and the shoulder girdle as a general warm-up and to reduce the hypertonicity of the muscles, paying specific attention to the deltoids, infraspinatus, teres group, pectoralis major, and biceps brachii.

2. Administer facilitated stretching of the rotator cuff muscle group. Stretching that follows the warm-up massage helps further reduce hypertonicity and eases the tension on the rotator cuff tendons.

3. Include more focused work to the muscle belly connected to the affected tendon. If accessible, the application of longitudinal stripping and pin-and-stretch strokes will further enhance the pliability of the muscles and reduce tension on the tendon attachment.

4. Position the athlete to provide access to the target tendon. Refer to the section earlier on tendon palpation for each of the cuff tendons.

   The initial application of DTF lasts about 1 minute using moderate pressure, that is, enough pressure to engage the tendon and "scrub" it against the bone. This may be somewhat painful for the athlete at the beginning, and the practitioner should adjust the pressure to keep the discomfort at about a 6 on a 10-point pain scale. Near the end of the first minute, the discomfort typically will have abated significantly. In some cases, it will remain the same, or it may increase.

5. After the first minute of DTF, the focus shifts to more general massage for the upper extremity and shoulder girdle, or perhaps to the uninvolved side, to give time for the treated tendon to rest.

6. Return to the affected area for another round of DTF. This time, the duration of treatment may be up to 3 minutes, as long as the discomfort rating is at or below a 6 on a 10-point scale.

7. Administer pain-free isolytic contractions to help reduce protective inhibition and help the muscles return to full activation.

8. Finish the treatment with another round of facilitated stretching for the cuff muscles.

9. Frequent application of ice is important to help control pain posttreatment.

10. Ideally, treatment is given every other day. Following the initial session, the friction portion of subsequent sessions can be longer (up to 9 minutes total) but still given in two or three doses per session. Each dose is given long enough for the pain to subside to near zero.

11. The total duration of treatment depends on the severity of the injury, the frequency of treatment, and the athlete's self-care activities.

Self-Care Options

If perpetuating factors are noted, these must be modified or eliminated to ensure that the injury does not reoccur. Once the tendon pain is eliminated, initiate a program of flexibility and progressive strengthening. If mobility has been limited as a result of pain, pendulum exercises, wall walking, and stick or towel exercises are all valuable for restoring pain-free ROM.

Because the main function of the rotator cuff is to stabilize the humerus in the glenoid fossa, strengthening work that focuses on scapular positioning and stability are appropriate. These would include isometrics, scapular squeezes, and resistance band work.

Case Study

Female Swimmer With Shoulder Pain Referred to Physician

The client is a 14-year-old female club volleyball player that had joined the school swim team (backstroke and fly stroke) five weeks prior to visit. Presented with right shoulder pain that reached a level 8 on a 0–10 scale when active, lowering to a level 3 with rest and ice. She had stopped swimming the day before initial visit.

Active and passive ROM assessment of right shoulder showed normal ROM in all movement planes of the shoulder except external rotation, but pain and weakness with all movement planes when performing resisted ROM. Unlike maintenance sessions of the past, participant could only tolerate very light pressure, and hypertonicity was found in numerous muscles of the shoulder joint and shoulder girdle. Main focus was on sedating the tissues with slow, steady, gentle strokes. Moist heat was applied to the affected area after assessment and treatment, but client showed little improvement. Recommended rest, contrast hydrotherapy and use of topical analgesic, and rescheduled for six days later.

Upon second visit, the athlete reported that she had spent two days in an arm sling, and had not participated in swimming or volleyball. Pain level was still at a high level, reported at a 6–7 when active. ROM and hypertonicity were similar to first visit. While starting treatment, she revealed that she had hit her head and jammed her neck two days prior to symptoms when she misjudged the distance of the pool wall and swam into it (she had not reported any neck discomfort). Active ROM of the neck revealed restriction in all movement planes of the neck except flexion. Extension was severely restricted. Treatment was immediately stopped, and the athlete was referred to her primary physician to evaluate neck trauma.

Upon examination by her physician, the athlete was diagnosed with assorted cervical issues due to the blunt force trauma of hitting the pool wall and was prescribed medications and physical therapy. Both the neck and the shoulder issues were resolved, and the athlete was able to successfully return to playing club volleyball. Both the athlete and her mother were very grateful for the referral.

Massage therapy is an effective healing modality, but to maintain professional integrity, it is just as important to know the appropriate time and be willing to refer out to other healthcare practitioners.

Kirk Nelson, CPNMT, BCTMB
Touchwork of Weston, Weston, MO

Triathlete With Painful Shoulder and Limited ROM

The client is a 59-year-old male triathlete. Five years ago he dislocated his left shoulder. For the past five years, the right shoulder has compensated for the left shoulder, leaving the right shoulder with limited range of motion. On initial assessment, the client was not able to actively abduct the right arm past 90° without pain and without moving his head forward and was restricted to approximately 155° of active abduction. Putting on a sweater or even a T-shirt caused pain and discomfort. Not only did he have difficulty raising his arm to the side, but he also had difficulty raising his arm forward.

Treatment occurred over a 6-week period in which effleurage and petrissage were introduced as general techniques to the following muscles and groups: scapular retractors, scapular protractors, rotator cuff, upper fibers of trapezius, deltoids, triceps, and biceps. As treatments progressed, more emphasis was placed on glenohumeral joint play and myofascial techniques. The glenohumeral joint received anterior and posterior grades 1 and 2 joint mobilizations along with humeral distraction. Muscles treated with pin and stretch included the pectoralis major, pectoralis minor, scalenes, sternocleidomastoid, levator scapulae, subscapularis, and latissimus dorsi. Also receiving treatment was the subclavius. To complement this treatment, the athlete was given a specific postural exercise for his home program. This simple exercise is performed by lowering the shoulder and shoulder blade, then bringing the shoulder blades together. By the sixth treatment, the client was able to wave to people without issue, but more importantly he competed in a Half Ironman triathlon with close to full range of motion at the shoulder.

Mike Grafstein, RMT, R.Kin, SMT(C), CAT(C)
Meridian Spine and Sport, Toronto, Canada

Tennis elbow (lateral epicondylitis) is the most common overuse injury of the elbow, resulting from repetitive strain to the common extensor tendons of the wrist. Although this condition is named for a sport in which it's common, it can also occur in other activities that involve repetitive stress on the wrist extensors.

Signs and Symptoms

Lateral epicondylitis (or epicondylosis if no inflammation is present) is characterized by a deep ache at the lateral epicondyle that is made worse by activity. Other symptoms may include pain at the lateral elbow, mild to moderate swelling, and limitation of wrist extension or flexion. The athlete may also experience sudden twinges of extreme pain. In well-advanced cases, sharp pain is often reported when gripping a racket or even shaking hands.

Typical History

Tennis elbow, like most overuse conditions, develops gradually over several months. It may flare up suddenly as a result of increased intensity of activity, such as competing in a tennis tournament. If the injury is not the result of a racket sport, look for repetitive motion in the client's daily activities.

Relevant Anatomy

In most cases, the primary injury is tendinopathy of the extensor carpi radialis brevis (ECRB) tendon, just distal to its attachment on the lateral epicondyle. The rest of the wrist and finger extensors may be affected by the presence of tennis elbow, either by becoming hypertonic or by becoming inhibited because of pain. See figure 7.12 for illustrations indicating the wrist and finger extensors.

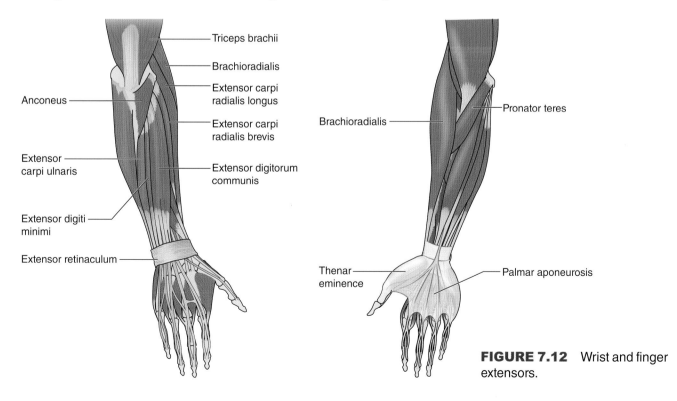

FIGURE 7.12 Wrist and finger extensors.

Extensor Carpi Radialis Brevis

The extensor carpi radialis brevis (ECRB) originates from the common extensor tendon at the lateral epicondyle of the humerus and inserts into the dorsoradial aspect of the base of the third metacarpal bone. Actions include extension of the wrist (with the ECR longus and ulnaris) and assisting radial deviation (abduction).

Extensor Carpi Radialis Longus

The extensor carpi radialis longus (ECRL) originates on the distal third of the lateral supracondylar ridge of the humerus, lying between the origin of the brachioradialis and the lateral epicondyle and inserts into the dorsoradial aspect of the base of the second metacarpal bone. Actions include extending the wrist (along with the ECR brevis and ulnaris) and assisting radial deviation (along with the flexor carpi radialis).

Supinator

The supinator originates from the posterior ulna, the lateral epicondyle, ligaments of the elbow and radioulnar joint, and the anterior capsule of the humeroulnar joint and inserts into the anterolateral aspect of the radius, just distal to the insertion of the biceps brachii. Actions include primary supinator of the hand and forearm; with the elbow flexed, the biceps brachii assists supination and assists elbow flexion when the hand is in neutral.

The radial nerve passes through the supinator muscle, and radial nerve entrapment may create symptoms similar to tennis elbow. Trigger points in the supinator may create referred pain that mimics tennis elbow and can be deactivated as part of the overall treatment for tennis elbow. Fun fact: Because supination is a stronger action than pronation, bolts and screws are designed to tighten by supination of the right forearm (righty-tighty, lefty-loosey).

Anconeus

The anconeus originates from the posterior aspect of the lateral epicondyle of the humerus and inserts into the lateral aspect of the olecranon process and the proximal posterior ulna. Actions include assisting triceps in extension of the elbow and assisting stabilization of the elbow joint during supination and pronation. The anconeus is thought to be secondarily involved in chronic cases of tennis elbow when additional stress placed on it results in compensation or inhibition of the extensor carpi radialis brevis.

Brachioradialis

The brachioradialis originates from the upper two-thirds of the supracondylar ridge of the humerus and inserts into the lateral radius, just proximal to the styloid process. Actions include flexion at the elbow, especially when the hand is in the neutral position; it may assist resisted pronation and supination. The brachioradialis may be secondarily involved with tennis elbow because of its proximity to the extensor carpi radialis longus.

Assessment

Observation

In severe cases, visible swelling over the lateral epicondyle may be present.

ROM Assessment

Active motion at the wrist consists of flexion, extension, abduction (radial deviation), and adduction (ulnar deviation). Depending on the severity of the injury, these motions may or may not cause pain. Passive motion is generally pain free except for wrist flexion, which may stretch painful tissues on the extensor side of the forearm, especially with the elbow extended.

Resisted extension of the wrist is painful. Resisted radial deviation may also be painful.

Manual Resistive Tests

The athlete, sitting or standing, places her wrist in neutral, forearm pronated. The examiner grasps the lateral elbow with one hand, and the other hand provides resistance as the athlete attempts to extend the wrist (see figure 7.13). This isometric contraction should begin slowly and build to a strong engagement of the target muscles. With the elbow flexed, the test will engage the ECR brevis more fully; with the elbow extended, the test will focus more on the ECR longus. Pain or weakness is a positive finding. Resisted extension of the middle finger (also known as Maudsley's test) is commonly positive for pain or weakness in tennis elbow (Fairbank and Corlett 2002) (see figure 7.14). If no pain occurs, the examination widens to include the other muscles that might cause lateral epicondyle pain, such as the supinator, brachioradialis, and anconeus.

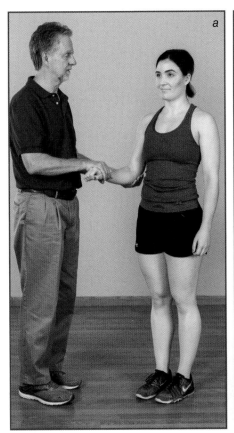
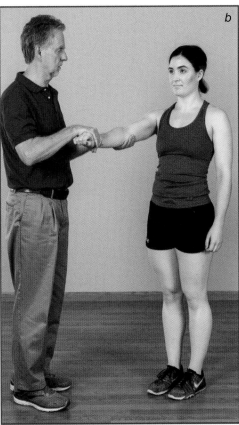

FIGURE 7.13 Resisted wrist extension test: with *(a)* elbow flexed and *(b)* elbow straight.

FIGURE 7.14 Middle-finger extension test.

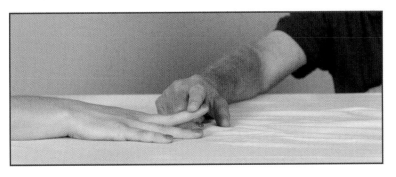

Precautions and Contraindications

Avoid palpatory or massage techniques that irritate the radial nerve.

Differential Diagnosis

Radial tunnel syndrome.

Palpation

Palpation over the lateral epicondyle should be done from the side, rather than from the top to avoid pressing into the brachioradialis, the supinator, and the radial nerve. Tenderness may be reported at the common extensor origin on the lateral epicondyle, the myotendinous junction of the ECR brevis, and the origin of the ECR longus on the supracondylar ridge. The site of maximal tenderness should correspond to the findings of the manual resistive tests.

Perpetuating Factors

In racket sports, improper form is the main factor contributing to tennis elbow. Poor form can result from inadequate conditioning that leads to fatigue of the torso and shoulder muscles, which puts additional stress on the forearm extensor muscles. Other factors to be investigated include biomechanical imbalances, scapular dyskinesis, repetitive motion, trigger points in associated muscles, and radial nerve entrapment.

Treatment Plan

Deep transverse friction is the centerpiece of treatment for tennis elbow that also includes soft tissue work on associated muscles that may contribute to the symptoms.

A typical treatment session is as follows:

1. Apply compressive effleurage and petrissage and broad cross-fiber work to the muscles of the forearm and upper arm as a general warm-up and to reduce the hypertonicity of the muscles.

2. Administer facilitated stretching of the wrist extensors. Stretching that follows the warm-up massage helps further reduce hypertonicity and eases the tension on the affected tendons.

3. Include more focused work to the belly of the muscle connected to the affected tendon. The application of longitudinal stripping and pin-and-stretch strokes will further enhance the pliability of the muscles and reduce tensile stress on the tendon attachment.

4. Administer DTF to the affected tendon transverse to the tendon fiber attachment direction as follows:

   - *ECR longus*: Because the tendon fibers attach perpendicular to the long axis of the humerus, friction is administered vertically along the humerus, just proximal to the supracondylar ridge (see figure 7.15).

   - *ECR brevis*: With the forearm nearly fully pronated, the myotendinous junction is directly over the radial head, and the friction is administered horizontally across either the epicondyle (origin) or the radial head (myotendinous junction) or both (see figure 7.16).

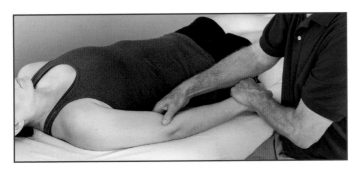

FIGURE 7.15 The path of the ECR longus causes its tendon to attach transversely on the humerus, so DTF is applied in a superior–inferior direction proximal to the supracondylar ridge.

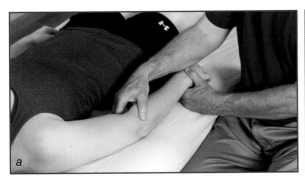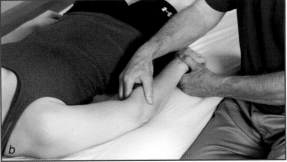

FIGURE 7.16 DTF for the ECR brevis is administered to *(a)* its epicondylar attachment or *(b)* its myotendinous junction, or both.

The initial application of DTF lasts about 1 minute using moderate pressure, that is, enough pressure to engage the tendon and "scrub" it against the bone. This may be somewhat painful for the athlete at the beginning, and the practitioner should adjust the pressure to keep the discomfort at about a 6 on a 10-point pain scale. Near the end of the first minute, the discomfort typically will have abated significantly. In some cases, it will remain the same, or it may increase.

5. After the first minute of DTF, the focus shifts to more general massage for the upper extremity and shoulder girdle, or perhaps to the uninvolved side, to give time for the treated tendon to rest.

6. Return to the affected area for another round of DTF. This time, the duration of treatment may be up to 3 minutes, as long as the discomfort rating is at or below a 6 on a 10-point scale.

7. Administer pain-free isolytic contractions to help reduce protective inhibition and help the muscles return to full activation.

8. Finish the treatment with another round of facilitated stretching for the extensor muscles.

9. Frequent application of ice is important to help control pain posttreatment.

10. Ideally, treatment is given every other day. Following the initial session, the friction portion of subsequent sessions can be longer (up to 9 minutes total) but still given in two or three doses per session. Each dose is given long enough for the pain to subside to near zero.

11. The total duration of treatment depends on the severity of the injury, the frequency of treatment, and the athlete's self-care activities.

Self-Care Options

If perpetuating factors are noted, these must be modified or eliminated to ensure that the injury does not reoccur. Once the tendinopathy pain is eliminated, initiate a program of flexibility and progressive strengthening.

Exercise and Flexibility Plan

To fully rehabilitate the muscles and tendons around the elbow, strengthening and flexibility work must begin when the client is pain free and before they return to the activity that caused the injury. Because tendons gain strength more slowly than muscles do, weight or resistance training should begin with minimal weight or resistance and high repetitions. Strengthening should be done in all ranges of motion at the forearm and wrist, with special attention given to eccentric exercise: flexion, extension, supination, pronation, radial deviation, and ulnar deviation. A regular program of facilitated stretching is also useful in maintaining maximum ROM.

Case Study

Elite Softball Pitcher With Multiple Diagnoses

At the time of this occurrence, the patient was an elite DI athlete. A multiple All-American and two-time Team USA member, she began her collegiate career as an overpowering softball pitcher. During the first three years of her career, she suffered a variety of musculoskeletal issues, mostly due to repetitive stress, in her right shoulder, arm, and forearm. A combination of sports massage and physical therapy resolved these complaints. In addition to these common complaints, she suffered a broken right ulna before her sophomore year, and was diagnosed with lumbar stenosis her junior year.

Her senior season was more challenging. Initially, she reported the usual complaints. However, by the third week of play, she began to complain of pain in her right neck, forearm, and hand, combined with a weakening grip. The pain and weakness worsened over the course of the season. Her grip strength, usually above 100 pounds, decreased to less than 40 pounds. She had difficulty straightening her elbow, and her forearm and hand began to swell. Over the course of that season, she was variously diagnosed with carpal tunnel syndrome, thoracic outlet syndrome, and exertional compartment syndrome (ECS) (mid-shaft fractures can contribute to ECS).

Initial treatment consisted of effleurage and petrissage to warm the muscles, followed by gentle, rhythmic compressions to assess the tissues. Assessment was followed by the Golgi tendon organ (GTO) technique to relax the affected muscles, then deep transverse friction to treat tight bands, and direct digital pressure to treat tender points. The involved tissues included anterior and middle scalenes, pectoralis minor, semispinalis cervicis, splenius capitis, and extensor digitorum. After ECS was diagnosed, we used gentle spreading strokes, combined with heat, to soften the fascia. This approach allowed her to pitch successfully into the postseason. She underwent carpal tunnel surgery after the season, allowing her to continue her career professionally.

Esteban A Ruvalcaba, LMT, BCTMB
Massage Therapies of Columbia, Columbia, MO

Golfer's elbow (medial epicondylitis or epicondylosis) is the same type of injury as tennis elbow, except it occurs at the attachment of the common flexor tendon on the medial epicondyle of the humerus. Although this condition is named for a sport in which it's common, the injury can also occur in other situations involving repetitive flexion of the wrist and fingers.

Signs and Symptoms

Medial epicondylitis (or epicondylosis if no inflammation is present) is characterized by a deep ache at the medial epicondyle, made worse by activity, especially any activity involving grip. Ulnar nerve symptoms (cubital tunnel syndrome) may also be present in up to 20% of cases (Kohn 1996).

Typical History

Golfer's elbow, like most overuse conditions, develops gradually over a period of several months. It may flare up suddenly as a result of increased intensity of activity, such as competing in a golf tournament. If the injury is not the result of golf, look for repetitive motion in the athlete's daily activities. The athlete may report painful limitation of wrist extension or flexion.

Relevant Anatomy

In most cases, the primary injury is tendinopathy of the common tendon of the wrist flexors at and just distal to the attachment on the medial epicondyle. See figure 7.17 for an illustration indicating the wrist and finger flexors.

Flexor Carpi Radialis

The flexor carpi radialis originates from the medial epicondyle of the humerus via the common flexor tendon and inserts into the base of the second and third metacarpals. Actions include wrist flexion (along with the flexor carpi ulnaris) and wrist abduction (with the extensor carpi radialis longus and brevis).

Flexor Carpi Ulnaris

The flexor carpi ulnaris originates from two heads: The humeral head attaches to the medial epicondyle by way of the common flexor tendon; the ulnar head originates from the medial aspect of the olecranon process and the proximal two-thirds of the posterior ulna. It inserts into the pisiform bone. Actions include wrist flexion (with the flexor carpi radialis) and wrist adduction (with the extensor carpi ulnaris). The ulnar nerve passes between the two heads of the flexor carpi ulnaris as it enters the forearm.

Flexor Digitorum Superficialis

The flexor digitorum superficialis originates from two heads. The humeroulnar head arises from the medial epicondyle via the common flexor tendon and from

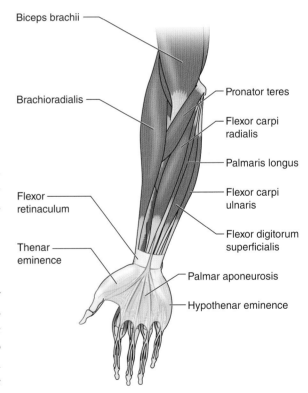

FIGURE 7.17 Wrist and finger flexors.

Biceps brachii

Brachioradialis

Flexor retinaculum

Thenar eminence

Pronator teres

Flexor carpi radialis

Palmaris longus

Flexor carpi ulnaris

Flexor digitorum superficialis

Palmar aponeurosis

Hypothenar eminence

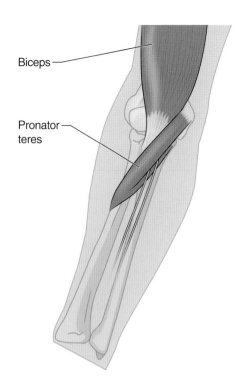

Biceps

Pronator teres

FIGURE 7.18   Pronator teres.

the medial aspect of the coronoid process, proximal to the pronator teres. The radial head originates from the radius, obliquely between the insertions of the biceps brachii and the pronator teres. The two heads are connected by a fibrous arch, through which pass the median nerve and the ulnar artery. It inserts into the middle phalanx of each finger. Actions include flexing the middle phalanges, then the proximal phalanges, as well as the hand at the wrist.

Palmaris Longus

The palmaris longus originates from the medial epicondyle and inserts into the palmar aponeurosis and the transverse carpal ligament. Actions include flexing the wrist and tensing the palmar aponeurosis. It may also assist pronation. The palmaris longus is often absent. The tendon of the palmaris longus lies superficial to the flexor retinaculum. When present, it can readily be seen when the palm is cupped and the wrist is flexed.

Pronator Teres

The pronator teres (see figure 7.18) originates from two heads. The main, humeral head attaches to the medial supracondylar ridge and the medial epicondyle. The small ulnar head attaches at the medial aspect of the coronoid process of the ulna. The muscle inserts into the midpoint of the lateral radius. Actions include assisting the pronator quadratus in pronation of the forearm and assisting flexion of the elbow against resistance. The median nerve enters the forearm between the two heads of the pronator teres.

Assessment

Observation

In severe cases, visible swelling over the medial epicondyle may be present.

ROM Assessment

Active motion at the wrist consists of flexion, extension, abduction (radial deviation), and adduction (ulnar deviation). Depending on the severity of the injury, these motions may or may not cause pain. Passive motion is generally pain free except during wrist or finger extension, which may stretch painful tissues on the flexor side of the forearm, especially with the elbow extended. Resisted flexion of the wrist is painful. Resisted ulnar and radial deviation and resisted pronation may also be painful.

Manual Resistive Tests

The athlete, sitting or standing, places the wrist in neutral, with forearm supinated. The examiner grasps the medial elbow with one hand, and the other hand provides resistance as the athlete attempts to flex the wrist (see figure 7.19). This

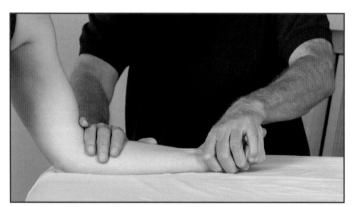

FIGURE 7.19   Resisted wrist flexion test for golfer's elbow.

isometric contraction should begin slowly and build to a strong engagement of the target muscles. Pain or weakness is a positive finding. If this test elicits no pain, the examination widens to include the other muscles that could cause medial epicondyle pain, such as the palmaris longus, pronator teres, and flexor digitorum superficialis.

Precautions and Contraindications

Avoid palpatory or massage techniques that irritate the ulnar or median nerve.

Differential Diagnosis

Cubital tunnel syndrome and ulnar collateral ligament injury.

Palpation

Once the functional assessment has narrowed the field of possible suspects, palpation of the common flexor tendon identifies the exact site at which deep transverse friction will be applied. Generally, the injury occurs either at the periosteal attachment to the epicondyle or at the myotendinous junction, which lies about .25 inch (6.3 mm) distal to the epicondyle (Cyriax 1993).

Perpetuating Factors

Training errors increase the risk of developing medial epicondylosis. Athletes typically report increased intensity or duration of activity before the onset of symptoms as well as a lack of adequate warm-up. Improper technique in golf or tennis is one of the major causes of medial epicondylosis. Equipment errors include the use of an incorrectly sized tennis racket or golf club grip. Functional risk factors include weakness, poor endurance, and poor flexibility of the forearm.

Treatment Plan

Deep transverse friction is the centerpiece of treatment for golfer's elbow. Treatment also includes soft tissue work on associated muscles that may contribute to the symptoms.

A typical treatment session is as follows:

1. Apply compressive effleurage and petrissage and broad cross-fiber work for the muscles of the forearm and hand as a general warm-up and to reduce the hypertonicity of the muscles.

2. Administer facilitated stretching of the wrist and finger flexors and the pronator teres. Stretching that follows the warm-up massage helps further reduce hypertonicity and eases the tension on the affected tendons.

3. Include more focused work to the belly of the muscles of the wrist and finger flexors. The application of longitudinal stripping and pin-and-stretch strokes will further enhance the pliability of the muscles and reduce tension on the tendinous attachment.

4. Position the athlete to administer DTF to the affected structures. The forearm is supported in full extension and supination, providing a bony foundation to "scrub" the tendon against. Friction is applied in a nearly horizontal direction, following the contour of the epicondylar ridge. DTF at the myotendinous junction is applied just distal to the epicondyle in a horizontal (anterior–posterior) direction (see figure 7.20).

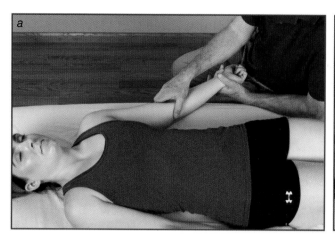 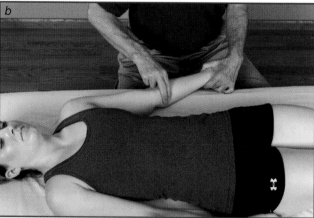

FIGURE 7.20   DTF for the common flexor tendon is administered *(a)* to its epicondylar attachment or *(b)* to its myotendinous junction, or both.

The initial application of DTF lasts about 1 minute using moderate pressure, that is, enough pressure to engage the tendon and "scrub" it against the bone. This may be somewhat painful for the athlete at the beginning, and the practitioner should adjust the pressure to keep the discomfort at about a 6 on a 10-point pain scale. Near the end of the first minute, the discomfort typically will have abated significantly. In some cases, it will remain the same, or it may increase.

5. After the first minute of DTF, the focus shifts to more general massage for the upper extremity and shoulder girdle, or perhaps to the uninvolved side, to give time for the treated tendon to rest.

6. Return to the affected area for another round of DTF. This time, the duration of treatment may be up to 3 minutes as long as the discomfort rating is at or below a 6 on a 10-point scale.

7. Administer pain-free isolytic contractions to help reduce protective inhibition and help the muscles return to full activation.

8. Finish the treatment with another round of facilitated stretching for the flexor muscles.

9. Frequent application of ice is important to help control pain posttreatment.

10. Ideally, treatment is given every other day. Following the initial session, the friction portion of subsequent sessions can be longer (up to 9 minutes total) but still given in two or three doses per session. Each dose is given long enough for the pain to subside to near zero.

11. The total duration of treatment depends on the severity of the injury, the frequency of treatment, and the athlete's self-care activities.

Self-Care Options

If perpetuating factors are noted, these must be modified or eliminated to ensure that the injury does not reoccur. Once the tendinosis pain is eliminated, initiate a program of flexibility and progressive strengthening.

Exercise and Flexibility Plan

To fully rehabilitate the muscles and tendons around the elbow, strengthening and flexibility work must begin when the athlete is pain free and before they return to the activity that caused the injury. Because tendons gain strength more slowly than muscles, weight or resistance training should begin with minimal weight and resistance and high repetitions. Strengthening should be done in all ranges of motion at the forearm and wrist, paying special attention to eccentric exercise: flexion, extension, supination, pronation, radial deviation, and ulnar deviation. Grip strength training should also be included. A regular program of facilitated stretching is also useful in maintaining maximum ROM.

Case Study

Female Yoga Practitioner With Shoulder Pain

The client was unsure when the initial injury occurred. She reported that it could have begun with a bike accident in 2013 or at martial arts training in 2016. She had a variety of treatments, including two steroid injections. She presented with restricted internal rotation and restricted abduction to 160°, all in the right shoulder. The right upper and middle trapezius, rhomboids, subscapularis, serratus anterior, anterior deltoid, pectoralis major, and infraspinatus were all hypertonic.

A variety of techniques were employed to treat the client, including general massage (petrissage, effleurage, kneading, and squeezing) to those areas aforementioned because the shoulder region was so generally hypertonic. As time went on, the tissues around the shoulder normalized and it became apparent that the central area of injury was the subscapularis. On closer inspection, the subscapularis had a scarred area in the superior aspect including the tendon. Active and passive pin-and-stretch techniques were used to soften the scarring and reintegrate it into the healthy tissue matrix. Scar tissue does not go away, but it can be softened and reintegrated into the non-affected tissue.

After six sessions, the client reported that the shoulder was operating at nearly 100% efficiency. She is participating in group fitness training and yoga. She can do the downward dog pose, which substantially loads the shoulder. She also has full abduction and substantially improved internal rotation. She wants to continue her recovery, and has begun resistance band exercises for the rotator cuff, which should lead to further improvement.

Charles McGrosky, CMT
Christchurch Therapeutic Massage Centre, Christchurch, New Zealand

Bicipital Tendinopathy

Bicipital tendinopathy is an overuse injury to the tendon of the long head of the biceps brachii. Biceps tendinopathy is rarely seen in isolation and often occurs concurrently with other shoulder injuries, such as rotator cuff pathologies, labral tears, and shoulder instability.

Signs and Symptoms

The most common symptom reported by athletes is a deep, throbbing ache at the front of the shoulder, exacerbated by pushing and pulling overhead or by lifting. Patient description of pain location is often vague (especially in low-level tendinosis). Pain may also refer down the arm to the deltoid insertion, and occasionally down to the hand in the radial distribution (Churgay 2009). An occasional snapping sound or sensation in the shoulder may be the result of the tendon subluxing from the bicipital groove secondary to rupture of the transverse humeral ligament (Gleason 2006). The most common physical sign for bicipital tendinopathy is tenderness to direct palpation at the bicipital groove.

Typical History

Bicipital tendinopathy is common in throwing sports and among swimmers and gymnasts. It's also common in weightlifting, bodybuilding, and some contact sports. Workers in occupations that involve overhead shoulder work or heavy lifting are also at risk.

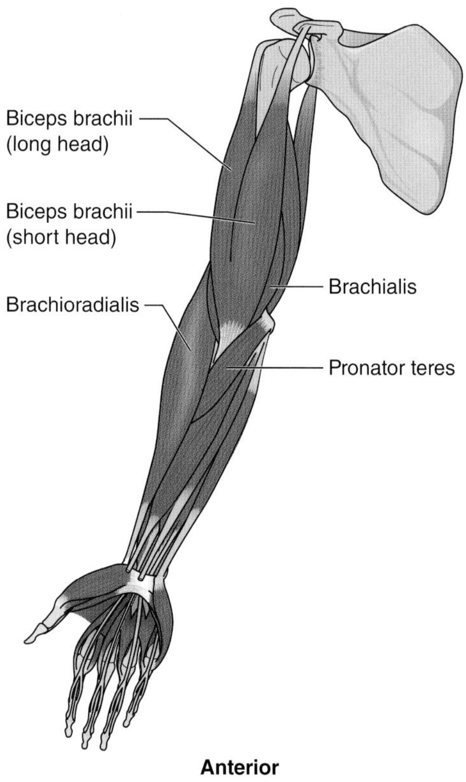

Relevant Anatomy

The biceps brachii muscle (see figure 7.21) consists of a short head and a long head that merge with one another to form the primary supinator and flexor of the forearm.

The tendon of the long head of the biceps arises from the supraglenoid tubercle and the superior glenoid labrum. The tendon travels obliquely inside the shoulder joint, passes across the anterior head of the humerus, and exits the joint within the bicipital groove, held in place by the transverse humeral ligament. The bicipital groove is formed by the greater tuberosity (lateral) and the lesser tuberosity (medial) of the humerus. The short head of the biceps arises from the coracoid process (often conjoined with the tendon of the coracobrachialis) and courses along the humerus medial to the long head of the biceps. The muscle bellies converge distally to form a tendon that inserts onto the radial tuberosity.

Although the biceps crosses both the shoulder and elbow joints, its main actions are elbow flexion and forearm supination. Wine lovers activate both these functions when opening a bottle with a corkscrew: The biceps brachii first unscrews the cork (supination), and then pulls the cork out of the bottle (flexion). The biceps also flexes the arm at the shoulder. Additionally, the long head of the biceps assists abduction of the humerus and acts strongly to help stabilize the humeral head, especially during abduction and external rotation. The short head assists adduction of the humerus.

Biceps brachii (long head)

Biceps brachii (short head)

Brachioradialis

Brachialis

Pronator teres

Anterior

FIGURE 7.21 Biceps brachii.

Assessment

Observation

Bicipital tendinopathy typically occurs along with other shoulder pathologies. Because biceps symptoms are similar to those of rotator cuff injuries and labral tears, isolating biceps issues during assessment can be challenging. If the transverse humeral ligament has ruptured, it may be possible to see or feel the biceps tendon subluxing out of the bicipital groove when the muscle is activated.

ROM Assessment

Because of the prevalence of concurrent impingement issues, ROM testing specifically for bicipital tendinopathy is not fruitful.

Manual Resistive Tests

In the Yergason's test, the athlete sits or stands with the arm at the side, elbow flexed to 90°, and the forearm pronated (see figure 7.22). The examiner sits or stands beside the athlete and provides resistance as the athlete attempts to supinate the forearm. Localized pain at the bicipital groove indicates a positive result.

Another test to verify this condition is the uppercut test, in which the athlete sits or stands with the arm at the side, elbow flexed to 90°, forearm supinated, and the hand closed into a fist. The examiner sits or stands beside the athlete and provides resistance as the athlete attempts to flex the arm upward, as if delivering a boxing uppercut (see figure 7.23). Localized pain or clicking at the bicipital groove indicates a positive result.

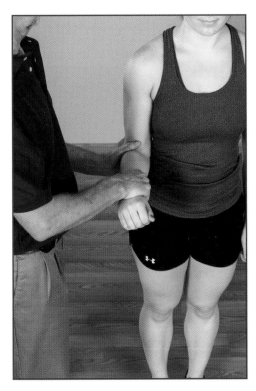

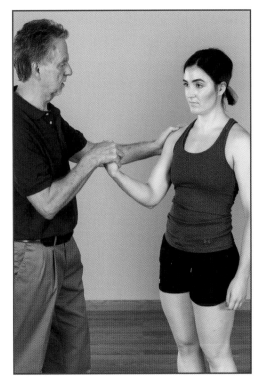

FIGURE 7.22 Yergason's test.

FIGURE 7.23 Uppercut test.

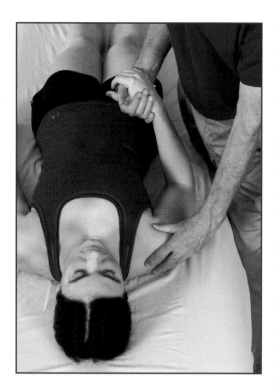

FIGURE 7.24 Palpation of bicipital groove.

Palpation

The palpatory exam provides the most accurate assessment of bicipital tendinopathy (Churgay 2009). Here, the athlete is supine on the treatment table, with the arm at the side and the hand resting on the anterior hip. This aligns the arm in about 10° of internal rotation, and the bicipital groove faces directly forward. The practitioner places the flat of the thumb or two fingers across the bicipital groove and, with moderate pressure, bends the athlete's elbow and passively rotates the humerus back and forth (see figure 7.24). Pain with this movement is positive for bicipital pathology.

Differential Diagnosis

Rotator cuff injury, labral injury, and shoulder impingement.

Perpetuating Factors

Bicipital tendinopathy is often accompanied and perpetuated by other conditions, including scapular dyskinesis (faulty scapular mechanics), rotator cuff impingement, or subacromial bursitis. Bicipital tendinopathy is also frequently exacerbated when the athlete returns to the precipitating activity too soon.

Treatment Plan

Deep transverse friction is the primary treatment for bicipital tendinopathy and can be sandwiched between preparatory strokes and finishing techniques. The severity of the condition and the length of time it's been present are both factors that influence recovery.

A typical treatment session is as follows:

1. Apply compressive effleurage and petrissage and broad cross-fiber work for the upper extremity and the shoulder girdle as a general warm-up and to reduce the hypertonicity of the muscles, paying specific attention to the biceps brachii.

2. Administer facilitated stretching of the biceps brachii. Stretching that follows the warm-up massage helps further reduce hypertonicity and eases the tension on the tendon.

3. Include more focused work to the muscle belly. The application of longitudinal stripping and pin-and-stretch strokes will further enhance the pliability of the muscle and further reduce tension on the tendon attachment.

4. Position the athlete to provide access to the tendon. This is the same position used for the palpation exam (see figure 7.25). The application of friction is accomplished by maintaining broad thumb or finger pressure against the bicipital groove and slowly rotating the humerus back and forth. This is typically more comfortable for the athlete than "digging in" by moving the thumb across the tendon.

The initial application of DTF lasts about 1 minute using moderate pressure, that is, enough pressure to engage the tendon and "scrub" it as the humerus rotates back and forth. This may be somewhat painful for the athlete at the beginning, and the practitioner should adjust the pressure to keep the discomfort at about a 6 on a 10-point pain scale. Near the end of the first minute, the discomfort typically will have abated significantly. In some cases, it will remain the same, or it may increase.

5. After the first minute of DTF, the focus shifts to more general massage for the upper extremity and shoulder girdle, or perhaps to the uninvolved side, to give time for the treated tendon to rest.

6. Return to the affected area for another round of DTF. This time, the duration of treatment may be up to 3 minutes as long as the discomfort rating is at or below a 6 on a 10-point scale.

7. Administer pain-free isolytic contractions to help reduce protective inhibition and help the muscle return to full activation.

8. Finish the treatment with another round of facilitated stretching for the biceps.

9. Frequent application of ice is important to help control pain posttreatment.

10. Ideally, treatment is given every other day. Following the initial session, the friction portion of subsequent sessions can be longer (up to 9 minutes total) but still given in two or three doses per session. Each dose is given long enough for the pain to subside to near zero.

11. The total duration of treatment depends on the severity of the injury, the frequency of treatment, and the athlete's self-care activities.

Self-Care Options

If perpetuating factors are noted, these must be modified or eliminated to ensure that the injury does not reoccur. Once the tendon pain is eliminated, initiate a program of flexibility and progressive strengthening. Because bicipital tendinopathy is a symptom of larger shoulder and rotator cuff issues, self-care should focus on restoring the pliability and strength of the static and dynamic stabilizers of the shoulder girdle and improving the shoulder's pain-free ROM.

Baseball Pitcher With Biceps Tendinopathy

The client is a 17-year-old male, right-handed baseball pitcher diagnosed with biceps tendinosis. He pitches for his high school baseball team and plays year-round in multiple offseason leagues. He was originally diagnosed by his physician with a strained rotator cuff in his right arm and completed physical therapy with no improvement. Upon further evaluation by the physician, he was re-diagnosed with biceps tendinosis. He has been unable to play baseball since the injury occurred while pitching in a game. He has significant pain with any rotation of the shoulder, particularly involving the overhand motion required for throwing. He also stated that he tends to sidearm his throws and that makes it hurt even more. Upon examination, he had limited ROM in his shoulder and severe pain with overhand movement. He also had minimal strength in his arm.

The client attended four treatments, each 30 minutes in length. Each session utilized several sports massage techniques that included warming up the shoulder soft tissues with compressive effleurage and petrissage, broad cross-fiber strokes of the distal attachment of the biceps, isolytic contractions of the biceps followed by active release techniques (ART) on any adhesions remaining in the affected tissues. After the initial visit, there were immediate improvements in range of motion with decreased pain. By the fourth visit, he had no pain and full range of motion in the shoulder.

Mary Riley, LMT
Riley Sports Massage, Cleveland, Ohio

Lacrosse Player with Rotator Cuff Injury

The client is a 19-year-old intercollegiate lacrosse player. He was initially diagnosed with a full tear of the infraspinatus and supraspinatus tendons. The infraspinatus was torn at the insertion of the muscle located at the greater tubercle of the humerus. The supraspinatus was torn at the insertion-located superior facet of the greater tubercle of the humerus. The two tendons were surgically reattached, and the patient was in a sling for 4 weeks post-surgery to include sleeping.

Post-surgical physical therapy included icing the shoulder 3 to 5 times (15 minutes each time) per day. Passive range of motion (ROM) of the glenohumeral joint. Neuromuscular electric stimulation (NMES) was used. Strength and stabilization exercises was implemented for the rotator cuff.

The client is 12 weeks post-surgery and has yet to attain a "normal" ROM of FF 140–150°, IR/ER 60°. The goal of the massage therapy is to improve ROM to considered norms and to prevent "frozen shoulder."

The initial massage therapy intake included passive, active ROM to assess baseline ROM. Active resisted testing used to determine the site of adhesions. Inflammation was not present at the time of intake.

Compressive effleurage/petrissage applied to prepare tissues. Both pin-and-stretch and neuromuscular therapy and multidirectional cross-fiber friction were applied to address superficial adhesions in soft tissue. Joint decompression was utilized to address adhesions within the joint capsule. The focus of the hands-on therapy was on surgically reattaching the musculature and compensating for the injury to include subscapularis, teres minor, medial deltoid, and upper trapezius.

Facilitated stretching and the application of contrast heat/cold therapy was incorporated to support hands-on work and improve flexibility. Sessions were set at 2 times a week for 30° for 3 weeks. Re-evaluated at session 6.

The client's ROM after eight sessions was effectively 145° FF, 70° IR, and 60° ER. Moved to 1 time a week for 2 weeks. Progressively moving to 1 time a month for 2 months.

George Glass, LMT, BCTMB, MEd
Glass & Glass Bodywork, Durango, CO

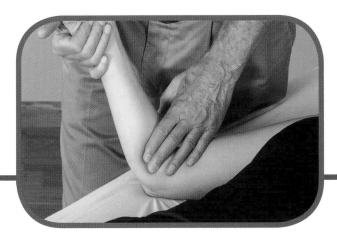

Chapter 8

Sports Massage for Nerve Entrapment Syndromes

The focus of this chapter is on nerve entrapment pathologies. These conditions are also referred to as nerve compression syndromes, compression neuropathy, and entrapment neuropathy. Nerves sustain injury primarily in three ways: through pressure (crush, compression and entrapment, repetitive stress), cuts and tears, and stretching and tension.

Nerve entrapment is usually defined as direct pressure on a single peripheral nerve. Symptoms of entrapment vary widely but typically include pain, tingling, numbness, and sometimes muscle weakness. According to Lowe (2016, para 9),

> Nerve compression injury occurs as a result of two main factors: force load and time. Force load is the amount of pressure applied to the nerve. Time refers to the amount of time that compressive load is applied. Note that significant nerve injury can occur with a very light force load if it is applied for a long time (like nerve compression in the wrist).

Symptoms can arise just from direct compression or may become apparent only when the nerve is subject to stress from being stretched while anchored in the soft tissues instead of being free to slide. This stretch-while-anchored situation is known as adverse mechanical tension or adverse neural tension. This excess tensile stress is thought to narrow the overall diameter of the nerve fiber, which then compresses the connective tissue components within the nerve (epineurium, perineurium, and endoneurium). These layers have their own nerve and nutrient supply and can be the source of symptoms when compromised (Lowe 2018).

Double crush syndrome, more accurately called double compression syndrome, refers to peripheral nerve compression in which there is proximal compression on a nerve bundle (e.g., at the nerve root or the thoracic outlet) and a second more distal compression (e.g., at the carpal tunnel). It's hypothesized that the proximal compression sensitizes the distal nerve so that relatively minor stress distally creates symptoms that would not normally occur if the proximal compression were not present.

When treating nerve compression syndromes, the therapeutic goal is to improve the pliability of the tissues that contribute to the entrapment, thereby reducing the compressive forces on the neural structures, allowing them to move more freely and to heal. As part of the assessment and treatment of nerve compression syndromes, nerve glides (also known as nerve flossing or nerve tension tests) can be used to test for restrictions in nerve mobility. When used for assessment, nerve glides are performed by carefully placing progressive tension on the nerve being tested. These nerve tension tests were first described by Elvey (1994) and have since been expanded and modified by numerous practitioners, most notably, the Australian physiotherapist David Butler (2000).

Nerve glide assessments are always performed on the unaffected side first to determine a baseline of normal movement. As with all special tests that have varying degrees of accuracy, nerve glide assessment is always used as part of a more thorough evaluation rather than as a stand-alone assessment. The same movements used to test for nerve mobility restrictions can be used to help restore normal nerve movement as part of a larger treatment program for entrapment pathologies.

Please note that other treatment approaches may also be appropriate for the injuries presented here. The suggested treatment progressions for each injury discussed in this chapter are the author's preferred approaches.

Quadrilateral Space Syndrome

The quadrilateral space, also known as quadrangular space, is located posterior and inferior to the glenohumeral joint and contains the axillary nerve and posterior humeral circumflex artery (see figure 8.1). Quadrilateral (quadrangular) space syndrome (QSS) is an entrapment pathology in which the axillary nerve and the posterior humeral circumflex artery are compressed as they pass through the space. Entrapment can be limited to just the nerve or the artery or can compromise both.

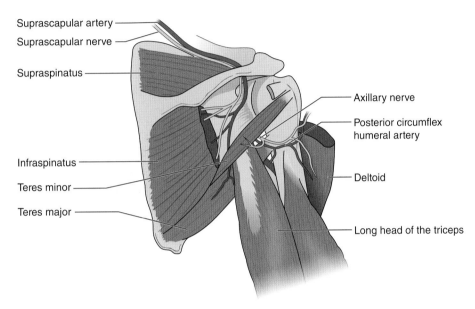

Suprascapular artery
Suprascapular nerve
Supraspinatus
Infraspinatus
Teres minor
Teres major
Axillary nerve
Posterior circumflex humeral artery
Deltoid
Long head of the triceps

FIGURE 8.1 The axillary nerve and posterior humeral circumflex artery travel through the quadrilateral space.

Signs and Symptoms

Dull, intermittent ache is common in the posterior and lateral shoulder, often worse at night, especially if the athlete sleeps on the affected shoulder. In throwing athletes, symptoms are worse with overhead activity or in the late cocking and acceleration phase of throwing (abduction and lateral rotation). According to Stecco, "These symptoms could also be due to an overuse syndrome, typical of overhead throwers, that causes a densification of the axillary fasciae" (Stecco 2015, p. 238). Point tenderness over the quadrilateral space is common, accompanied by referred pain into the deltoid. Atrophy or weakness of the teres minor and deltoid muscle may be present, leading to weak external rotation of the humerus. Paresthesia may be reported in the sensory distribution of the axillary nerve over the deltoid muscle in the lateral shoulder and upper posterior arm (see figure 8.2).

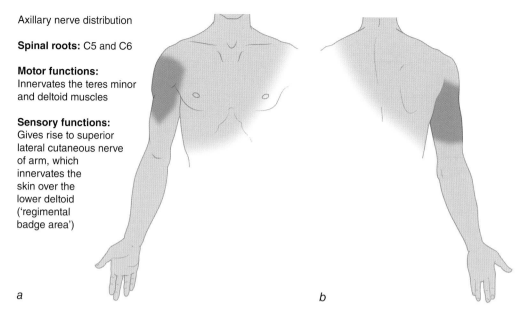

Axillary nerve distribution

Spinal roots: C5 and C6

Motor functions:
Innervates the teres minor and deltoid muscles

Sensory functions:
Gives rise to superior lateral cutaneous nerve of arm, which innervates the skin over the lower deltoid ('regimental badge area')

a   *b*

FIGURE 8.2   The axillary nerve sensory distribution to the skin over the inferior two-thirds of the deltoid muscle, also called the "regimental badge" area.

Typical History

This is considered to be a rare condition but is included here because the author has treated several cases in overhead athletes. QSS typically occurs in the dominant shoulder of athletes 20 to 40 years of age and predominantly in males. QSS may be incorrectly attributed to subacromial impingement or other shoulder conditions because many of the symptoms overlap. Fibrous bands in the soft tissues, which may be the fascial densification noted by Stecco, are typically implicated in QSS. Funk (n.d.) reports that paralabral cysts secondary to tears of the inferior labrum are also a common cause of QSS, especially in athletes who participate in contact sports.

Common factors that contribute to QSS include the repetitive motion of overhead sports (swimming, basketball, volleyball) as well as poor throwing mechanics in baseball. Additional factors may include compression from carrying a heavy backpack, upward pressure into the quadrilateral space (for instance, improper crutch use), trauma from a fall on the shoulder, shoulder dislocation, and humeral fracture.

Relevant Anatomy

The quadrilateral space is a compartment formed by the teres minor superiorly, the teres major inferiorly, the long head of the triceps medially, and the surgical neck of the humerus laterally. Note that the teres minor is separated from the teres major by the tendon of the long head of the triceps as it passes through to its attachment on the infraglenoid tubercle. See figure 8.1.

Assessment

Investigation of this condition can be challenging because the symptoms of QSS mimic symptoms of other shoulder conditions, such as thoracic outlet syndrome, subacromial impingement, bursitis, and rotator cuff tear. QSS is typically diagnosed only after these other more common conditions have been misdiagnosed and treated.

Observation

In chronic cases, visible atrophy of the teres minor and deltoid muscles may be present.

ROM Assessment

Normal ROM is usually available at the shoulder, but abduction and external rotation (especially if performed together, as in a throwing motion) may be weak or re-create the athlete's symptoms. Horizontal adduction or internal rotation of the humerus may also be painful because these motions may tug on the entrapped axillary nerve.

Nerve Glide Assessment

A nerve glide movement can be used to assess the ability of the nerve to move through the quadrilateral space. This assessment is performed carefully to generate slight tension, but not to the point of discomfort. In this version of the nerve glide assessment, the athlete stands with shoulders relaxed, slightly bends the elbow, and slowly internally rotates the humerus, feeling for slight tension but not pain (see figure 8.3a). If this position is comfortable, the athlete depresses the shoulder, then laterally flexes the neck away from the shoulder (see figure 8.3b). Tension along the nerve distribution (especially into the deltoid) is normal; pain is not. If pain begins, ask the athlete to pinpoint the location because this will help isolate the location of the nerve entrapment.

Manual Resistive Tests

Resisted abduction and resisted external rotation may be weak and typically exacerbate the athlete's symptoms.

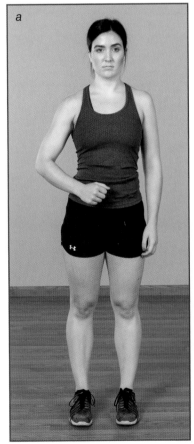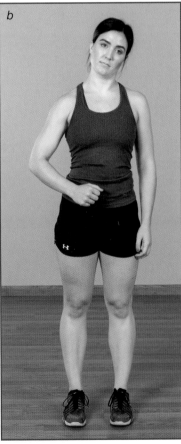

FIGURE 8.3   Nerve glide assessment for the axillary nerve. *(a)* Standing with shoulders relaxed, elbow bent and humerus internally rotated, feeling for slight tension. *(b)* Increase tension by depressing the shoulder and laterally flexing the neck.

Palpation

Careful palpation will reveal point tenderness in the quadrilateral space (see figure 8.4). Tenderness may also be reported with palpation over the anterior shoulder as well as the deltoid.

Fibrous bands are often present in the soft tissues of the quadrilateral space. According to Brown and colleagues (2015, p. 390),

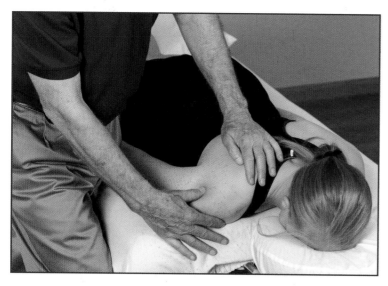

FIGURE 8.4 Palpation of the quadrilateral space may find point tenderness.

In cadaveric shoulder dissections, fibrous bands were located between the teres major and the long head of the triceps; external rotation reduced the cross-sectional area of the QS. The fibrous band often results from overt or occult repeated microtrauma to connective tissue in the QS with the formation of permanent scarring and adhesions.

The teres minor and major, the long head of the triceps and the posterior deltoid may be "ropey" or congested when palpated. Palpation may also exacerbate the athlete's symptoms, indicating the likely location of the nerve entrapment.

Precautions and Contraindications

Care must be taken when palpating for and treating nerve compression syndromes to avoid further irritating the already compromised neural structures.

Differential Diagnosis

Thoracic outlet syndrome, referred pain from neck structures, rotator cuff syndrome, and impingement syndrome.

Perpetuating Factors

Because QSS is typically the result of repetitive abduction and external rotation of the affected shoulder during sport or work activity, it's imperative to reduce these activities as much as possible during treatment.

Treatment Plan

The overall goal for treatment is to reduce the compression on the axillary nerve and restore pain-free motion in external rotation and abduction.

A typical treatment session is as follows:

1. Apply compressive effleurage and petrissage and broad cross-fiber work to the upper extremity and the shoulder girdle as a general warm-up and to reduce the hypertonicity of the muscles, paying specific attention to the deltoids, infraspinatus, and teres group.

2. Administer facilitated stretching of the rotator cuff muscle group. Stretching that follows the warm-up massage helps further reduce hypertonicity and tension in the shoulder girdle.

3. Apply longitudinal stripping and pin-and-stretch strokes to the teres minor, teres major, triceps, and deltoid muscles.

4. If fibrous bands are identified within or between the quadrilateral space muscles, the careful application of pain-free transverse friction will improve the pliability of these tissues. The initial application of DTF lasts about 1 minute using moderate pressure, as long as there is no increase in symptoms. During subsequent sessions, DTF may be administered for up to 3 minutes.

5. Administer pain-free isolytic contractions to the teres group, triceps, and posterior deltoid to help reduce protective inhibition and help the muscles return to full activation.

6. Finish the treatment with another round of facilitated stretching for the treated muscles.

Self-Care Options

If perpetuating factors are noted, these must be modified or eliminated to ensure that the injury does not reoccur. Once the symptoms have abated, initiate a program of flexibility and progressive strengthening. Focus on facilitated stretching into horizontal adduction and internal rotation and strengthening of the rotator cuff, deltoids, and triceps. Nerve glides are included to help the nerve continue to move freely though the quadrilateral space as it heals.

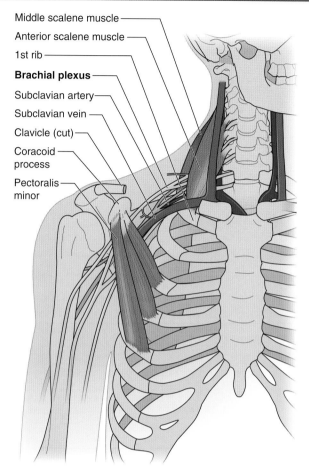

Middle scalene muscle
Anterior scalene muscle
1st rib
Brachial plexus
Subclavian artery
Subclavian vein
Clavicle (cut)
Coracoid process
Pectoralis minor

FIGURE 8.5 The brachial plexus is a neurovascular bundle that courses from the cervical spine through the chest and into the arm.

Thoracic outlet syndrome (TOS) describes a group of disorders that result from the compression, injury, or irritation of neurovascular structures (brachial plexus) in the thoracic outlet, which includes the region bordered by the scalene muscles (interscalene triangle), the first rib and clavicle (costoclavicular space) and the coracoid process, the pectoralis minor, and the underlying ribs (subpectoral space) (see figure 8.5).

Thoracic outlet syndrome typically manifests as pain, tingling, numbness, or pins and needles along the pathway of the brachial plexus. Additional symptoms may include weakness in the upper extremity, as well as color and temperature changes in the hand of the affected side. The three main manifestations of TOS follow:

1. *Neurogenic TOS* is the most common form of the condition and is more common in women. Bony or soft tissues in the lower neck and upper chest compress and irritate the nerves of the brachial plexus.

2. *Arterial TOS* is caused by impingement of the subclavian artery by bony or soft tissues.

3. *Venous TOS* is caused by impingement of the subclavian vein. This vein does not pass through the scalenes, so it is not affected by anterior scalene syndrome. The condition develops suddenly, often after unusual and tiring exercise of the arms.

Signs and Symptoms

Neurogenic TOS

The signs and symptoms of neurogenic TOS are pain, tingling, prickling, numbness, and weakness in the neck, chest, and arms and weakness or numbness of the hand (especially the fourth and fifth fingers). In chronic cases, hand muscles on the affected side may atrophy.

Arterial TOS

The signs and symptoms of arterial TOS are poor blood circulation to the arms, hands, and fingers, leading to cold sensitivity in the hands and fingers; pale skin caused by lack of arterial blood flow; and numbness, pain, or soreness in the fingers.

Venous TOS

The signs and symptoms of venous TOS are swollen veins in the anterior chest wall; swelling of the hands, fingers, and arms, accompanied by bluish or purple skin (caused by congestion of venous blood flow); and heaviness and weakness of the neck and arms.

Typical History

Because thoracic outlet syndrome is a multifaceted condition that manifests in a variety of ways, there is no typical history of onset. Factors that might contribute to the onset include the following:

- Sports that require repetitive motions that place the shoulder at the extreme of abduction and external rotation (such as swimming, baseball, volleyball, racket sports)
- Cervical flexion–extension injury (whiplash)
- Repetitive stress injury, especially from sitting at a keyboard for long hours
- Scalene hypertrophy (often seen in baseball pitchers)
- Postural factors (such as slumped or rounded shoulders, head forward)

Relevant Anatomy

TOS typically occurs at one or more common entrapment sites. The brachial plexus can be subject to excessive compression as it exits the cervical spine and passes between the anterior and middle scalenes (anterior scalene syndrome), as it crosses between the first rib and the clavicle (costoclavicular syndrome), and as it passes between the pectoralis minor and the underlying rib cage (pectoralis minor syndrome) (see figure 8.6). In fewer than 1% of the population, a cervical rib at C7 may be present that creates compression on the brachial plexus.

Because TOS is a multifaceted condition, it's useful to discuss the anatomy of the three main areas where it occurs.

Anterior Scalenes Entrapment Area

When the anterior and middle scalenes are hypertonic, they can compress the brachial plexus as it passes between them, causing symptoms of neurogenic or arterial TOS, but not the venous manifestation because the subclavian vein joins the brachial plexus inferior to the scalenes. The anterior scalene originates from the anterior aspect of the transverse processes of C3-6 and inserts onto the superior aspect of the first and second ribs. The middle scalene originates from the posterior aspect of the transverse processes of C2-7 and inserts onto the superior aspect of the first rib, lateral to the anterior scalene.

When the anterior and middle scalenes are acting unilaterally, they laterally flex and rotate the cervical spine to the same side. When they are acting bilaterally, they assist flexion of the cervical spine and also help stabilize the spine against lateral movement. The scalenes are traditionally ascribed an accessory respiratory function as they assist forced inspiration or "panic breathing" into the upper chest by elevating the first and second ribs. In recent years, improved electromyography studies have shown that the

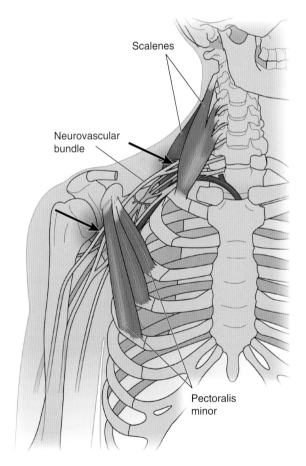

Scalenes

Neurovascular bundle

Pectoralis minor

FIGURE 8.6 The three common entrapments sites for TOS are at the scalene muscles, between the clavicle and first rib, and beneath the pectoralis minor.

scalenes are active even during quiet breathing. This has led some researchers to drop the accessory label and regard them as primary muscles of inspiration (Shurygina 1999).

Costoclavicular Entrapment Area

In this manifestation of TOS, the neurovascular bundle (including the nerve complex, the brachial artery, and the subclavian vein) is compressed as it passes between the first rib and the clavicle. Any of the three types of TOS may result from costoclavicular entrapment of the brachial plexus. Compression in this region is often attributed to slumping posture that causes the upper trunk to round forward and down, the shoulders to round forward into protraction, and the arms to medially rotate. This posture results in the clavicle pressing against the first rib, closing the costoclavicular space and compressing the neurovascular bundle. Additional factors may be a hypertonic subclavius muscle or scalene muscles elevating the first rib against the clavicle. A previously fractured clavicle may have a bony callus present that narrows the costoclavicular space.

The subclavius originates from the first rib and its cartilage and inserts onto the inferior surface of middle-third of the clavicle. Actions include drawing the clavicle inferiorly and anteriorly. It also assists in shoulder depression and may assist elevation of the first rib.

Pectoralis Minor and Rib Cage Entrapment Area

As the brachial plexus passes between the pectoralis minor and the underlying ribs (second, third, and fourth), a shortened pectoralis minor muscle can narrow this subpectoral space, compressing the neurovascular bundle, especially during hyperabduction of the arm, where the bundle can also press against the coracoid process. Any of the three types of TOS can occur from compression of the brachial plexus here.

The pectoralis minor originates from the third, fourth, and fifth ribs, near the costal cartilage and inserts on the medial and superior aspect of the coracoid process of the scapula. It stabilizes the scapula when the arm is exerting downward pressure (crutch walking, push-ups). When hypertonic, it may cause the inferior border of the scapula to wing out, and it also contributes to forward and rounded shoulders.

Assessment

A thorough evaluation helps to determine the likely location of the nerve entrapment and guide the possible treatment options.

Observation

Postural issues are often cited as factors in the development of TOS. A head-forward, slumping posture may contribute to compression of the brachial plexus. Examine skin color and temperature because arterial and venous TOS often cause abnormal skin color and temperature, especially in the hand. Also, atrophy of the hand muscles on the affected side may be observable.

ROM Testing

Limited lateral cervical flexion may indicate hypertonic scalene muscles. This is significant if on the affected side. Slumped posture, as well as pain, may limit shoulder flexion, abduction, and horizontal abduction.

Nerve Glide Assessment

Nerve glide exercise is used to assess the ability of the neurovascular bundle to move through the thoracic outlet. Perform this assessment carefully to generate slight tension, but not to the point of discomfort, and perform it first on the unaffected side. Nerve glides provide insight into possible entrapments but are just one piece of a larger evaluation process that must be carried out before determining what and where to treat.

Upper-Limb Tension Test

The upper-limb tension test (ULTT), also called the upper-limb neurodynamic test (ULNT), was developed by the late Robert Elvey, an Australian physiotherapist, author, and lecturer who pioneered and developed evaluation and treatment techniques in the field of neural mobilization (1994). This test is used to screen for sensitized nerves in the cervical spine, brachial plexus, and upper extremity but is not specific for one area.

In this version of the ULTT, the athlete plays an active part, rather than having the test administered passively. Performing the test this way permits both upper extremities to be tested simultaneously and uses the asymptomatic side as a control compared to the symptomatic side. Once symptoms appear, there is no need to continue the test (Sanders, Hammond, and Rao 2007). The positions are as follows:

1. The athlete abducts both arms to 90°, with the elbows straight (see figure 8.7a).

2. If no symptoms appear in position 1, the athlete extends both wrists (see figure 8.7b).

3. If no symptoms appear in position 2, the athlete slowly and carefully tilts the head first to one side, ear to shoulder, then to the other side (see figure 8.7c). Positions 1 and 2 are expected to elicit symptoms on the symptomatic side, and position 3 is expected elicit symptoms when the head is tilted to the contralateral, pain-free side as tension is applied to the brachial plexus. Pain down the arm, especially around the elbow or paresthesia in the hand or both is a positive result and indicates compression of the brachial plexus in one of three areas: the cervical spine, the scalene muscles, or the pectoralis minor.

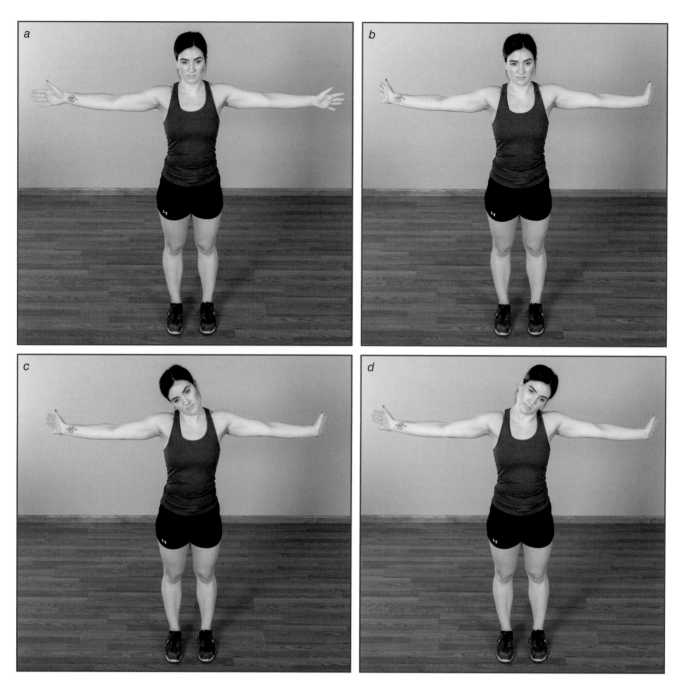

FIGURE 8.7 Upper Limb Tension Test (ULTT): *(a)* bilateral abduction of the arms to 90° for position 1, *(b)* add wrist extension for position 2, and *(c)* add cervical lateral flexion toward the affected side, and *(d)* away from the affected side.

Special Tests

Several positional tests have been developed to help identify TOS in general and to help pinpoint the location of the compression.

Roos Test

This test is also known as the elevated arm stress test (EAST test of Roos) and the 90° abduction in external rotation (90° AER) stress test. To perform the test, the patient elevates the arms in a "stick-em-up" or "I surrender" position (see figure 8.8). This test is positive for TOS with a reproduction of the athlete's symptoms of pain and paresthesia within 60 to 90 seconds but does not necessarily show a reduction of the radial pulse.

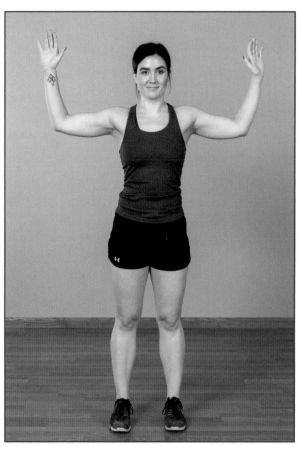

FIGURE 8.8　Roos test.

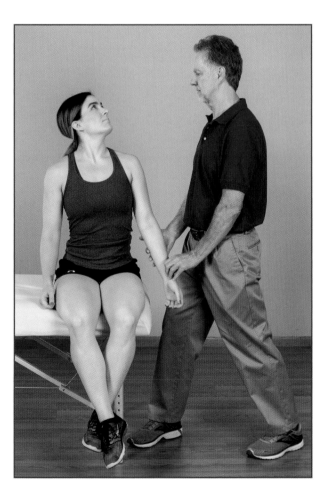

FIGURE 8.9　Adson's test.

Adson's Test

The athlete is seated with arms hanging at the sides and the examiner palpates the radial pulse. The athlete rotates the head toward the affected side and tilts the chin up while the examiner continues to monitor the radial pulse (see figure 8.9). The athlete accentuates the test by taking and holding a deep breath (scalenes are respiratory muscles). Loss or decrease in the strength of the radial pulse is a positive finding for anterior scalene syndrome.

Eden's Test

The athlete is seated with arms hanging down and the examiner palpates the radial pulse. The athlete pulls the shoulder girdle back and down and pushes the chest forward (military posture), while the examiner continues to monitor the radial pulse (see figure 8.10). The athlete accentuates the test by taking and holding a deep breath (lifts ribs tighter against clavicle). Loss or decrease in the strength of the radial pulse is a positive finding for costoclavicular syndrome.

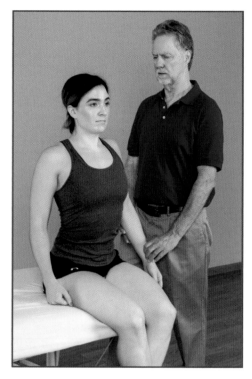

FIGURE 8.10   Eden's test.

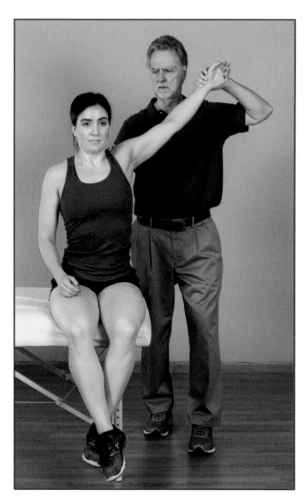

FIGURE 8.11   Wright's test.

Wright's Test

The athlete is seated with arms hanging down and the examiner palpates the radial pulse. The examiner passively moves the athlete's arm up and back into hyperabduction and external rotation, supporting the posterior shoulder girdle with one hand while continuing to monitor the radial pulse with the other hand (see figure 8.11). The athlete accentuates the test by taking and holding a deep breath (lifts rib cage tighter against the stretched pectoralis minor). Loss or decrease in the strength of the radial pulse is a positive indicator for pectoralis minor syndrome.

Precautions and Contraindications

Care must be taken when palpating for and treating nerve compression syndromes to avoid further irritating the already compromised neural structures.

Differential Diagnosis

Cervical radiculopathy, cervical or thoracic disc herniation, and clavicle injury.

Palpation

The results of the special tests and the nerve glide evaluation can be used to help guide the palpatory examination. Careful palpation is conducted first at the suspected area of neural compression. The soft tissues in the region around the entrapment are commonly hypertonic, stiff, or ropey. Neural symptoms may also be exacerbated by palpatory pressure, in which case the examiner moves the contact immediately.

Perpetuating Factors

As noted earlier, postural imbalances are thought to be key factors in the development and the perpetuation of TOS. Sports participation as well as daily activities also contribute to and perpetuate TOS and must be modified, at least for the period of treatment and rehabilitation.

Treatment Plan

The overall goal for treatment is to reduce the compression on the brachial plexus by reducing hypertonicity in the soft tissues as well as to help correct postural issues and to address muscle imbalances that contribute to the narrowing of the thoracic outlet causing the nerve compression.

A typical treatment session is as follows:

1. Apply compressive effleurage and petrissage and broad cross-fiber work to the neck, the shoulder girdle, and the upper extremity as a general warm-up and to reduce the hypertonicity of the muscles, paying specific attention to the scalenes, the sternocleidomastoid, the upper trapezius, and the pectoralis major.

2. Administer facilitated stretching of the scalenes, sternocleidomastoid, and the pectoralis major. Stretching that follows the warm-up massage helps further reduce hypertonicity and eases the tension in these muscles.

3. Include more focused work in the area identified as the site of nerve compression as follows:

   - *Anterior scalene syndrome.* The application of specific cross-fiber strokes, longitudinal stripping, and pin-and-stretch techniques will improve the pliability of the muscles. Follow this with another round of facilitated stretching.

   - *Costoclavicular syndrome.* Because hypertonic scalenes will elevate the ribs and contribute to the narrowing of the costoclavicular space, use the same protocol outlined in the previous bullet point to help normalize scalene tone and texture. Add pin and stretch and facilitated stretching for the subclavius muscle.

- *Pectoralis minor syndrome.* Once the pectoralis major has been relaxed in steps 1 and 2, pain-free palpation of the pectoralis minor through the major is possible. Administer specific cross-fiber strokes and pin-and-stretch techniques to improve the pliability of the pectoralis minor muscle belly. Follow this with facilitated stretching.

4. Have the athlete carefully perform the ULTT on the affected side and compare results to the initial assessment. If improvement is noted, repeat the ULTT several times as a therapeutic nerve glide, just until tension is felt. If the treatment helped reduce TOS symptoms, repeat it every 2 to 3 days to keep progressing toward full resolution. If the treatment was not successful the first time, try it again in 2 or 3 days. If there is still no improvement, shift the focus of treatment to other structures or to a different method of treatment.

Self-Care Options

If perpetuating factors are noted, these must be modified or eliminated to ensure that the injury does not reoccur. As pain diminishes, initiate a program of flexibility and progressive strengthening. The ULTT can be used as a self-care exercise to help maintain nerve mobility. Pain-free facilitated stretching is recommended to restore normal tone to hypertonic muscles, typically upper trapezius, levator scapulae, scalenes, sternocleidomastoid, pectoralis major, and pectoralis minor. Once pain free, the athlete can begin strengthening exercises for the scapular retractors and stabilizers.

Carpal tunnel syndrome (CTS) is a compression neuropathy of the median nerve as it passes under the transverse carpal ligament of the hand. This condition is the most commonly diagnosed upper-extremity nerve compression disorder in the United States and other developed countries. CTS appears to be closely associated with tenosynovitis of the flexor tendons in the carpal tunnel. The double crush phenomenon may also play a role in sensitizing the median nerve at the carpal tunnel.

Signs and Symptoms

At the wrist, the median nerve is composed of more than 90% sensory fibers (see figure 8.12). In CTS, the sensory fibers are the primary source of symptoms. These symptoms include paresthesia, numbness, and aching or burning pain in the sensory distribution of the hand and fingers (the palmar aspect of the thumb, the first to the inside of the fourth fingers, the palm, and the dorsal aspect of the first to the inside of the fourth fingers from MIP joint to the end of the fingers).

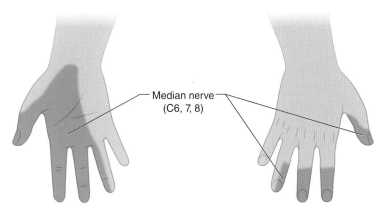

FIGURE 8.12 Median nerve sensory distribution.

In the early stages of CTS, symptoms are usually intermittent and occur with certain activities such as reading a book, knitting, and keyboarding. A classic manifestation of CTS is night symptoms that wake the athlete, especially if symptoms dissipate by shaking the hand and wrist. This may be caused by the common practice of sleeping with the wrists flexed. Athletes also often report weakness and clumsiness in the hand, making it difficult to perform fine movements such as buttoning a shirt or operating a zipper. Another common symptom is dropping objects held in the hand, such as a coffee cup. This is likely caused more by numbness leading to a loss of proprioception in the hand than by loss of motor control.

Carpal tunnel syndrome does not typically exhibit sensory loss over the thenar eminence of the hand. This is because the palmar cutaneous nerve serves that area and branches off the median nerve proximal to and passes over the carpal tunnel (see figure 8.13). This feature of the median nerve can help separate carpal tunnel syndrome from thoracic outlet syndrome or pronator teres syndrome.

Typical History

CTS is a syndrome affected by many and varied factors. Except in cases of acute trauma, CTS symptoms usually begin gradually, with no specific injury. Many clients re-

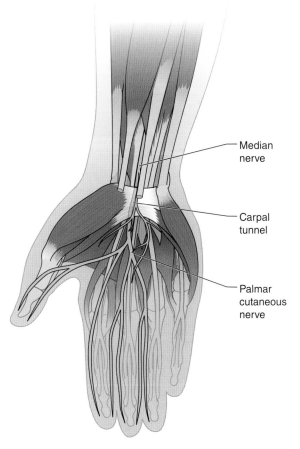

FIGURE 8.13 Palmar cutaneous nerve.

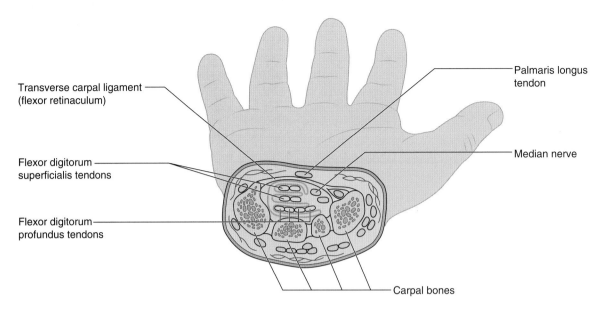

Transverse carpal ligament (flexor retinaculum)

Flexor digitorum superficialis tendons

Flexor digitorum profundus tendons

Palmaris longus tendon

Median nerve

Carpal bones

FIGURE 8.14   Carpal tunnel.

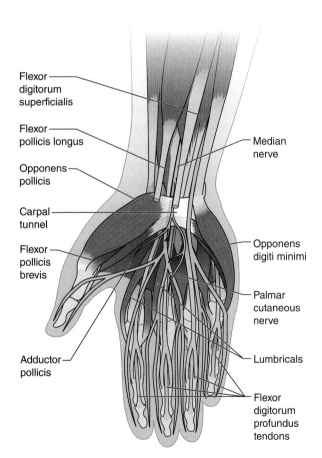

Flexor digitorum superficialis

Flexor pollicis longus

Opponens pollicis

Carpal tunnel

Flexor pollicis brevis

Adductor pollicis

Median nerve

Opponens digiti minimi

Palmar cutaneous nerve

Lumbricals

Flexor digitorum profundus tendons

FIGURE 8.15   The nine tendons that course through the carpal tunnel along with the median nerve are protected by synovial sheaths.

port that their symptoms come and go at first. As the condition worsens, symptoms occur more frequently and last longer before diminishing. In addition, work or athletic activities that may contribute to CTS (particularly in combination) include prolonged, severe force through the wrist; prolonged, extreme posture of the wrist; a large number of repetitive movements through the wrist and hand; and exposure to vibration and cold (Ashworth 2018).

Relevant Anatomy

The carpal tunnel floor and sides are formed by the carpal bones of the wrist, and the roof of the tunnel is formed by the transverse carpal ligament (also known as the flexor retinaculum). The tunnel contains the median nerve and nine sheathed tendons. These include the flexor pollicis longus, the four slips of flexor digitorum superficialis, and the four slips of flexor digitorum profundus (see figure 8.14). Because the carpal tunnel has little ability to expand, if the synovial sheaths become inflamed (tenosynovitis), they swell and create undue pressure against the median nerve, generating the symptoms of CTS (see figure 8.15). Additionally, repetitive activities may irritate the nerve.

Assessment

A thorough evaluation helps to determine whether the presenting symptoms are likely to be caused by median nerve entrapment at the wrist and guide the possible treatment options.

Observation

The wrist can be observed for swelling, excessive warmth or coolness, and discoloration. Atrophy in the muscles of the thenar eminence may be visible (see figure 8.16).

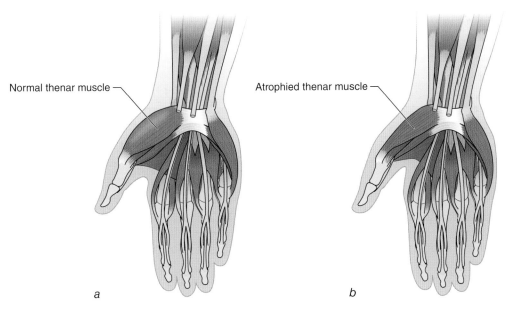

Normal thenar muscle

Atrophied thenar muscle

a

b

FIGURE 8.16 *(a)* Normal thenar eminence versus *(b)* atrophy of the thenar eminence which may occur in carpal tunnel syndrome.

ROM Assessment

Flexion and extension of the wrist and fingers may be limited because of pain.

Manual Resistive Tests

Weakness or atrophy in the hand muscles innervated by the median nerve may be present.

Abductor Pollicis Brevis Test

The athlete sits comfortably with the hand resting on the table, palm up, thumb in neutral. The athlete attempts to abduct (raise) the thumb perpendicular to the palm as the examiner applies downward pressure to the end of the thumb (see figure 8.17). This test isolates the abductor pollicis brevis. Weakness is considered a positive result.

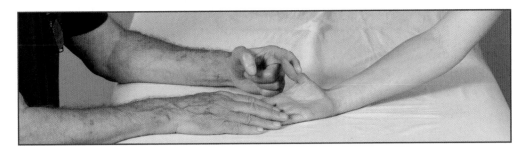

FIGURE 8.17 Abductor pollicis brevis resisted test.

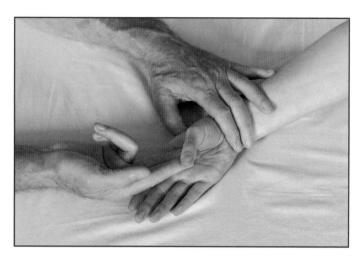

FIGURE 8.18   Flexor pollicis brevis resisted test.

Flexor Pollicis Brevis Test

The athlete sits comfortably with the hand resting on the table, palm up, thumb in neutral. The athlete attempts to flex the whole thumb toward the palm as the examiner resists the movement (see figure 8.18). This test isolates the flexor pollicis brevis, and weakness is considered a positive result.

Nerve Glide Assessment

This assessment is used to evaluate the ability of the median nerve to move freely through the carpal tunnel. Perform this assessment carefully to generate slight tension but not to the point of discomfort. In this version of the nerve glide assessment, the athlete stands with shoulders relaxed and spine lengthened. The arm is flexed to about 90°, and the wrist is extended. The thumb and first two fingers are extended, but the ring and little finger are relaxed (see figure 8.19a). This position targets (biases) the median nerve. If this position is comfortable, the athlete slowly lowers the arm, maintaining the extension on the wrist and fingers (see figure 8.19b). From here, the athlete slowly internally rotates the humerus, then slowly abducts the arm (see figure 8.19c). If at any point, pain or paresthesia in the median distribution is felt, the assessment is considered positive for median nerve involvement and stops.

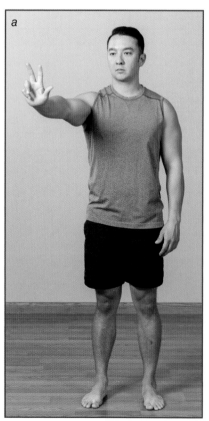
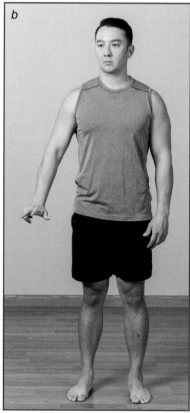
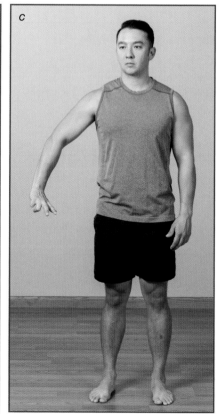

FIGURE 8.19   Median nerve glide assessment.

Special Tests

The following additional stress tests are often used as part of a thorough evaluation.

Phalen's Test

This test strongly compresses the median nerve within the carpal tunnel. The athlete presses the back of the hands together to flex the wrists to approximately 90° (see figure 8.20). If pain, paresthesia, or numbness in the median nerve distribution is reproduced within about 60 seconds, the test is considered positive.

Reverse Phalen's Test

This assessment increases tension on the median nerve as it crosses the wrist. The athlete presses the palms of the hands together to extend the wrists to approximately 90°, similar to a prayer position (see figure 8.21). If pain, paresthesia, or numbness in the median nerve distribution is reproduced within about 60 seconds, the test is considered positive.

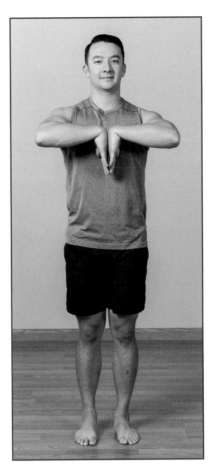

FIGURE 8.20   Phalen's test.

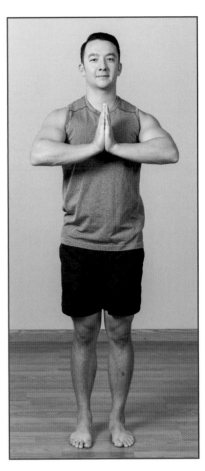

FIGURE 8.21   Reverse Phalen's test.

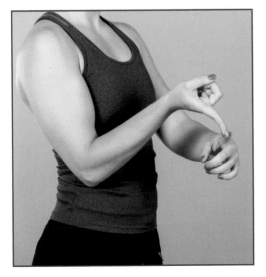

FIGURE 8.22   Tethered median nerve test.

Tethered Median Nerve Test

This test is useful in detecting chronic, low-grade median nerve compression. The athlete hyperextends the supinated wrist and the index finger for up to 1 minute (see figure 8.22). This position produces the greatest amount of distal nerve excursion through the carpal tunnel. Re-creation of symptoms is considered a positive result.

Tinel's Sign

The examiner performs light percussion over the median nerve as it passes under the transverse carpal ligament (see figure 8.23). Although this is the least sensitive of the median nerve tests, it is the most specific test for median neuropathy at the carpal tunnel. If this test elicits tingling or paresthesia in the median nerve distribution, it's considered positive.

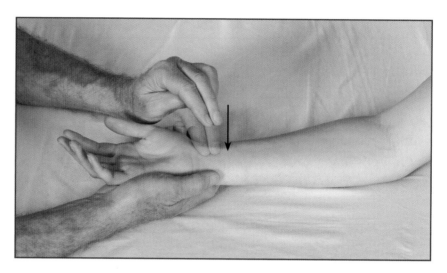

FIGURE 8.23 Tinel's sign.

Palpation

Careful palpation throughout the hand, wrist, and forearm will often reveal tenderness across the wrist, especially at the transverse carpal ligament, and may elicit an increase in symptoms. In chronic cases, the thenar eminence may be flaccid, indicating muscle atrophy. The wrist and finger flexors in the forearm may feel ropey or congested.

Precautions and Contraindications

Care must be taken when palpating for and treating nerve compression syndromes to avoid further irritating the already compromised neural structures.

Differential Diagnosis

Acute compartment syndrome, cervical disc compromise, diabetic neuropathy, and thoracic outlet syndrome.

Perpetuating Factors

Carpal tunnel syndrome can be caused and perpetuated by many factors related to the use of the hands and arms. Changing the pattern of use by reducing the frequency or intensity of the offending activities is critical during the healing process.

Treatment Plan

The overall goal for treatment is to reduce the compression on the median nerve and restore pain-free motion at the wrist and fingers.

A typical treatment session is as follows:

1. Apply compressive effleurage and petrissage and broad cross-fiber work to the upper extremity as a general warm-up and to reduce the hypertonicity of the muscles, paying specific attention to the wrist and finger flexors, the pronator teres, and the hand.

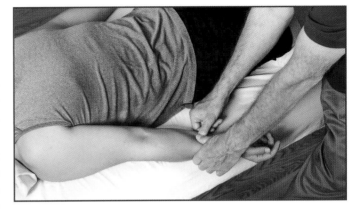

2. Administer facilitated stretching of the wrist and finger flexors. Stretching that follows the warm-up massage helps further reduce hypertonicity and tension in the forearm.

3. Apply longitudinal stripping to the wrist flexors (see figure 8.24) and pin-and-stretch strokes to the wrist flexors (see figure 8.25) and the pronator teres (see figure 8.26).

FIGURE 8.24   Longitudinal stripping for the wrist flexors.

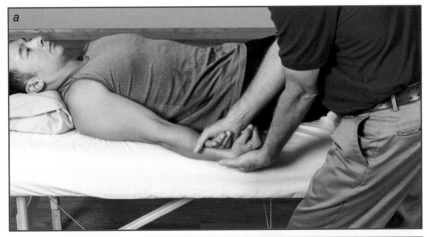

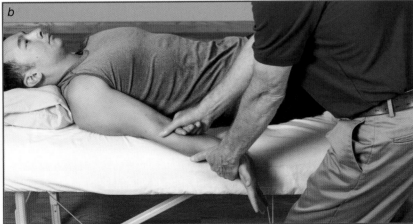

FIGURE 8.25   Pin and stretch for the wrist flexors: *(a)* starting position with the wrist and fingers flexed and *(b)* ending with the wrist and fingers extended.

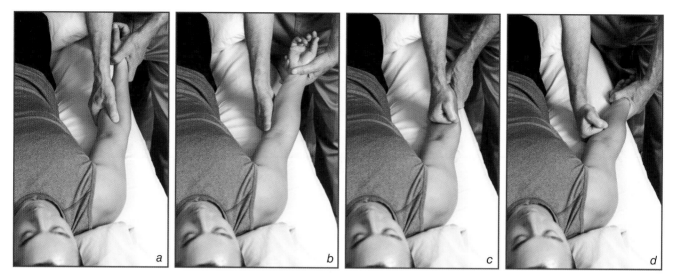

FIGURE 8.26 Pin and stretch for the pronator teres: *(a)* using the thumb, starting position with the forearm in neutral; *(b)* using the thumb, ending with the forearm supinated; *(c)* using a loose fist, starting position with the forearm in neutral; *(d)* using a loose fist, ending with the forearm supinated.

4. Use moderate-pressure transverse friction work to address muscles and tendons and to mobilize areas where the median nerve may be trapped in or between these tissues. Start with general friction to the muscle bellies of the wrist and finger flexors, performing more detailed work as fibrous bands are palpated (see figure 8.27). Use the fingers or the thumb to apply moderate-pressure transverse friction to the tendons at the wrist (see figure 8.28). Sheathed tendons, like those at the wrist, are held on a slight stretch as friction is applied perpendicular to the tendon fibers. Administer friction to the transverse carpal ligament, also perpendicular to the direction of the fibers.

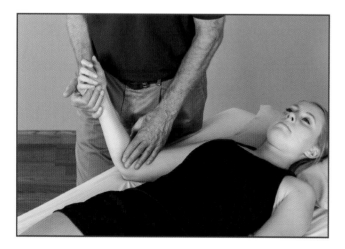

FIGURE 8.27 Transverse friction to fibrous bands in the forearm.

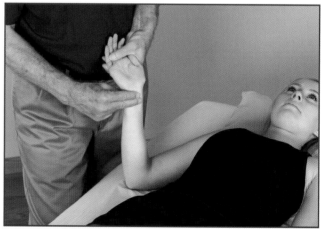

FIGURE 8.28 Transverse friction to sheathed flexor tendons, with the wrist slightly extended.

5. Administer pain-free isolytic contractions to the wrist flexors to help reduce protective inhibition and help the muscles return to full activation.

6. Finish the treatment with another round of facilitated stretching for the treated muscles.

Self-Care Options

If perpetuating factors are noted, these must be modified or eliminated to ensure that the injury does not reoccur. Once the symptoms have abated, initiate a program of flexibility and progressive strengthening. Focus on facilitated stretching for the wrist flexors and extensors and the pronator teres, accompanied by strengthening exercises for the wrist flexors and extensors. Nerve glides help the median nerve continue to move freely though the carpal tunnel as it heals.

Case Study

Golfer with Carpal Tunnel Syndrome

This client is a 54-year-old male, right-handed, golfer diagnosed with carpal tunnel syndrome. He has experienced numbness and tingling in both wrists for the last 12 months with the right wrist being more severe. The pain radiates up his arm on bad days. He stated that he first felt the pain come on while lifting weights. He is also an architect that spends most of his workday on the computer. After time off, he continued to work out and golf, but the pain and symptoms continued to increase, and he was unable to continue sports activities or work.

Upon examination, he had decreased ROM and pain in both wrists. He also had full numbness in the right hand and partial numbness in the left hand. He had minimal strength and wasn't able to pick up objects with the right hand.

In order to relieve tension through the carpal tunnel, several soft-tissue techniques were utilized. The goals of the treatments were to release any adhesions of the transverse carpal ligament and flexor retinaculum, to decrease the tension of all flexor muscles in the forearm, and to ensure there were no adhesions or muscle tension along the median nerve all the way up the arm.

Client attended 3 treatments, each 30 minutes. Each treatment utilized several sports massage techniques that included warming up the muscles of the arm with compressive effleurage and petrissage, longitudinal stripping and isolytic contractions of the forearm flexors, and active release techniques (ART) on any adhesions remaining. After the initial visit, there were immediate improvements in ROM of the wrist with decreased pain and numbness on both hands. By the third visit, all feeling had returned, there was no pain, and strength was improved.

Mary Riley, LMT
Riley Sports Massage, Cleveland, Ohio

Cubital Tunnel Syndrome

The cubital tunnel, near the medial elbow, is formed by the two heads of flexor carpi ulnaris (FCU). Cubital tunnel syndrome, also called ulnar neuropathy, is compression of the ulnar nerve as it passes through the cubital tunnel. It is the second most common nerve entrapment condition of the upper extremity, carpal tunnel syndrome being the most common. A related ulnar compression syndrome is commonly called cyclist's palsy or handlebar palsy because it often affects long-distance road cyclists or mountain bikers. In this condition, the ulnar nerve is compromised at Guyon's canal (formed by the pisiform and hamate bones of the wrist) by the prolonged pressure and vibration of holding the handlebars.

Signs and Symptoms

As with most nerve entrapment conditions, the typical symptoms of cubital tunnel syndrome include pain, paresthesia, and a burning sensation along the ulnar nerve distribution (see figure 8.29). Pain is generally reported more in the arm, up to and including the elbow area (see figure 8.30). Weakness in the fifth finger and ulnar side of the fourth finger and numbness in the dorsal ulnar aspect of the hand and fingers are also common. Symptoms may be exacerbated by prolonged elbow flexion during activities such as holding a phone to the ear or sleeping with a flexed elbow.

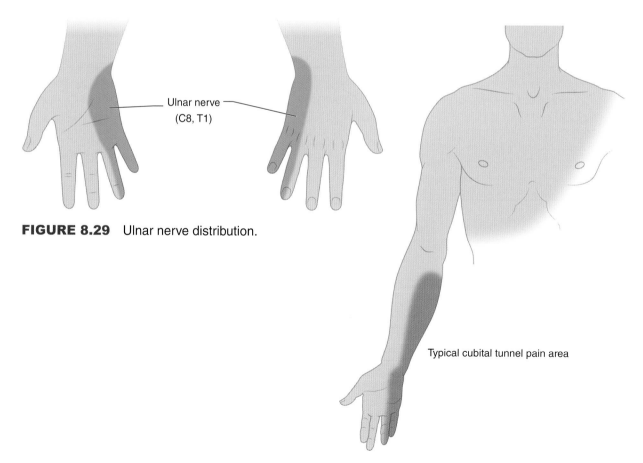

Ulnar nerve
(C8, T1)

FIGURE 8.29   Ulnar nerve distribution.

Typical cubital tunnel pain area

FIGURE 8.30   Typical cubital tunnel pain area.

Typical History

Cubital tunnel syndrome is typically considered a repetitive stress injury, associated with work or leisure activities. It's more common in clients whose work involves protracted periods of elbow flexion, such as holding telephones or carrying heavy trays of food or drink. Elbow flexion with the elbow pressed against a hard surface (leaning on a desk) increases the risk of this condition, most likely because of the increased intraneural pressure on the ulnar nerve in this position. According to Cutts,

> The American and Japanese literature places a heavy emphasis on the susceptibility of baseball throwers to cubital tunnel syndrome. Ulnar nerve symptoms during that part of the throwing cycle that involves extreme flexion (late cocking, early acceleration) is strongly suggestive of cubital tunnel syndrome. (Cutts 2007, p. 29)

The repetitive nature of other activities, such as swinging a hammer or playing the violin, may also lead to increased risk for developing cubital tunnel syndrome.

Relevant Anatomy

The cubital tunnel is the pathway at the elbow for the ulnar nerve. The floor of the tunnel is formed by the medial collateral ligament, the olecranon, and the joint capsule, and the roof of the tunnel is formed by the two heads of flexor carpi ulnaris and Osborne's ligament (see figure 8.31). One head of the FCU blends with the flexor tendon attachments at the medial epicondyle of the humerus, and the other attaches to the olecranon process of the ulna. They're connected by an aponeurosis (Osborne's ligament or the arcuate ligament of Osborne). The ulnar nerve passes through this tunnel to enter the forearm and must be able to both stretch and slide when the elbow bends. Sliding plays the greatest role in this process, although the nerve itself can stretch by up to .2 inches (5 mm) (Cutts 2007). Cutts also states that "In addition, the shape of the tunnel changes from an oval to an ellipse with elbow flexion. This manoeuvre also narrows the canal by 55%. Elbow flexion, wrist extension and shoulder abduction increases intraneural pressure by six times" (Cutts 2007, p. 28).

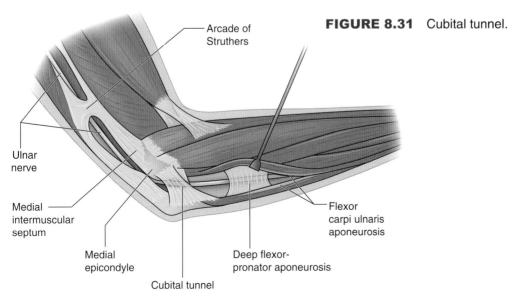

FIGURE 8.31   Cubital tunnel.

Arcade of Struthers

Ulnar nerve

Medial intermuscular septum

Medial epicondyle

Cubital tunnel

Deep flexor-pronator aponeurosis

Flexor carpi ulnaris aponeurosis

Although the ulnar nerve is subject to entrapment at six locations along its course through the arm, the cubital tunnel is by far the most common (see figure 8.32). The other five sites of potential ulnar nerve entrapment include the arcade of Struthers, the medial intermuscular septum, the medial epicondyle, the deep flexor pronator aponeurosis (between the heads of the flexor carpi ulnaris) and Guyon's canal.

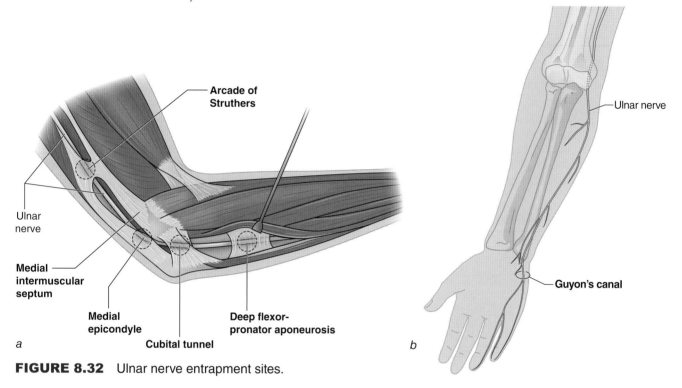

FIGURE 8.32 Ulnar nerve entrapment sites.

Assessment

A thorough evaluation helps to determine whether the presenting symptoms are likely to be caused by ulnar nerve entrapment at the cubital tunnel and guide the possible treatment options.

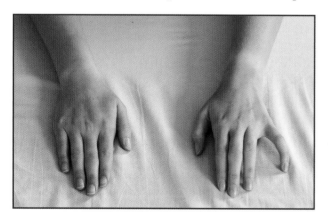

FIGURE 8.33 Wartenberg's sign, abduction and extension of the little finger, is caused by unopposed action of the extensor digiti minimi.

Observation

In chronic cases, clawing of the ring and little finger may be visible, along with atrophy of the web space between the thumb and index finger. When muscles innervated by the ulnar nerve are compromised, the little finger may be abducted and extended (muscles innervated by the intact radial nerve), which is called Wartenberg's sign (see figure 8.33). The client may complain of catching the finger when trying to put the hand in a pants pocket.

ROM Assessment

Flexion and extension of the wrist and fourth and fifth fingers may be limited by pain.

Manual Resistive Tests

Handshake Test

Cubital tunnel syndrome is often accompanied by motor symptoms that manifest as weakness in gripping. A simple handshake, comparing the affected and unaffected side, may reveal general weakness in the symptomatic hand.

Froment's Sign

This test assesses the grip strength between the thumb and index finger, accomplished by contraction of the adductor pollicis (adducting the thumb) and the first dorsal interosseous muscle (abducting the index finger). To perform the test, the examiner asks the client to hold a piece of paper between the thumb and index finger. The examiner then attempts to pull the object out of the client's hand. If the adductor pollicis is weak because of ulnar nerve injury, the client will experience difficulty maintaining the grip and will compensate by engaging the flexor pollicis longus to flex the thumb at the distal interphalangeal joint to maintain grip pressure (see figure 8.34).

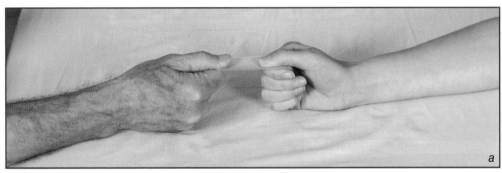

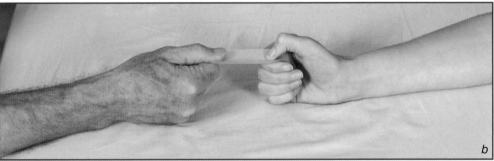

FIGURE 8.34   Froment's sign: *(a)* normal grip strength and *(b)* positive Froment's due to weakness of adductor pollicis.

Nerve Glide Assessment

This assessment is used to evaluate the ability of the ulnar nerve to move freely through the cubital tunnel. Perform this assessment carefully to generate slight tension, but not to the point of discomfort. In this version of the nerve glide assessment, the athlete stands with shoulders relaxed and spine lengthened, raises her arm to about 90° with the elbow straight, and extends the ring and little finger. The thumb and first two fingers are relaxed. This position targets (biases) the ulnar nerve. If this position does not create symptoms, the athlete slowly lowers the arm, fully flexing the elbow and keeping the wrist and fingers extended (see figure 8.35a). This "waiter's position" may compress the ulnar nerve at the cubital tunnel while maintaining some stretch across the wrist. If symptoms appear in 30 to 60 seconds, the test is positive. If no symptoms appear, the test may continue with the athlete maintaining wrist and elbow position and abducting the arm (see figure 8.35b). If at any point, pain or paresthesia in the median distribution is felt, the assessment is considered positive for ulnar nerve involvement and stops.

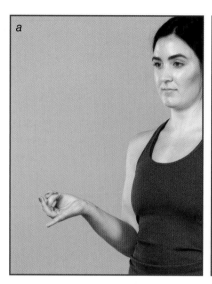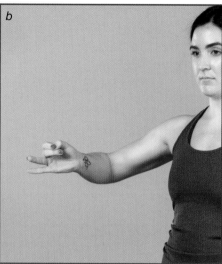

FIGURE 8.35 Ulnar nerve glide assessment: *(a)* standing relaxed, lower the arm to the side, fully flex the elbow, and keep the wrist and last two fingers extended. The thumb and first two fingers are relaxed. *(b)* To add more tension to the ulnar nerve, keep the same elbow, wrist, and finger positions, and abduct the arm.

Palpation

Careful palpation will often reveal point tenderness at the medial elbow, typically about an inch (2.5 cm) distal to the medial epicondyle. Palpation across the ulnar side of the wrist may also elicit an increase in symptoms. The wrist and finger flexors, especially the flexor carpi ulnaris, in the forearm may feel ropey or congested.

Precautions and Contraindications

Care must be taken when palpating for and treating nerve compression syndromes to avoid further irritation of the already compromised neural structures.

Differential Diagnosis

Cervical disc compromise, thoracic outlet syndrome, carpal tunnel syndrome, and epicondylitis.

Perpetuating Factors

Cubital tunnel syndrome can be caused and perpetuated by many factors related to the use of the hands and arms. Changing the pattern of use by reducing the frequency or intensity of the offending activities is critical during the healing process.

Treatment Plan

The overall goal for treatment is to reduce the compression on the ulnar nerve and restore pain-free movement and strength to the wrist and fingers.

A typical treatment session is as follows:

1. Apply compressive effleurage and petrissage and broad cross-fiber work to the upper extremity as a general warm-up and to reduce the hypertonicity of the muscles, paying specific attention to the wrist and finger flexors, the pronator teres, and the hand.

2. Administer facilitated stretching of the wrist and finger flexors. Stretching that follows the warm-up massage helps further reduce hypertonicity and tension in the forearm.

3. Administer longitudinal stripping (see figure 8.36) and pin-and-stretch strokes (see figure 8.37) to the wrist flexors, with focus on the flexor carpi ulnaris.

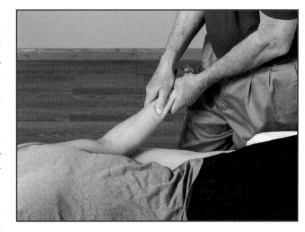

FIGURE 8.36   Longitudinal stripping to the flexor carpi ulnaris.

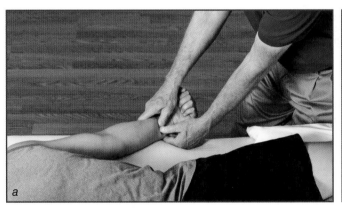

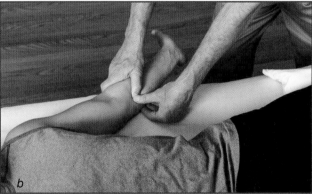

FIGURE 8.37   Pin and stretch of the flexor carpi ulnaris: *(a)* starting position with the wrist and fingers flexed and *(b)* ending with the wrist and fingers extended.

4. Use moderate-pressure transverse friction work to specifically address the flexor carpi ulnaris muscle belly to mobilize areas where the ulnar nerve may be trapped in or between these tissues (see figure 8.38).

5. Administer pain-free isolytic contractions to the wrist and finger flexors to help reduce protective inhibition and help the muscles return to full activation.

6. Finish the treatment with another round of facilitated stretching for the treated muscles.

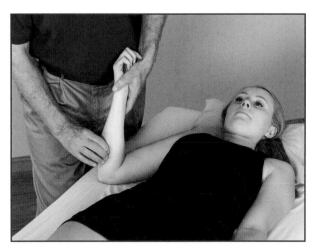

FIGURE 8.38   Transverse friction for the muscle belly of the flexor carpi ulnaris (FCU).

Self-Care Options

If perpetuating factors are noted, these must be modified or eliminated to ensure that the injury does not reoccur. Once the symptoms have abated, initiate a program of flexibility and progressive strengthening. Focus on facilitated stretching for the wrist flexors and extensors and the pronator teres, accompanied by strengthening exercises. Nerve glides help the nerve continue to move freely though the cubital tunnel as it heals.

Tarsal tunnel syndrome is a compression or traction neuropathy of the tibial nerve (or its branches) as it passes through the tarsal tunnel on the medial side of the ankle (see figure 8.39). Tarsal tunnel syndrome may occur with, or is often misdiagnosed as, plantar fasciitis or heel spurs.

Signs and Symptoms

Tarsal tunnel syndrome typically manifests with pain, tingling, or pins and needles along the medial aspect of the ankle and into the foot, especially the big toe, consistent with the tibial nerve distribution (see figure 8.40). Burning pain may also be reported at night or after long periods of standing, walking, or running. During the early stages of tarsal tunnel syndrome, the symptoms may be intermittent, then become more constant as the compression on the nerve gets worse. In advanced cases, there may be weakness in the toe flexors.

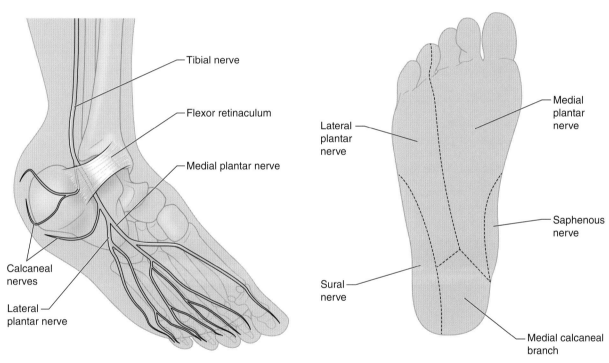

FIGURE 8.39 Tibial nerve and its branches: calcaneal, medial plantar, and lateral plantar.

FIGURE 8.40 Tibial nerve distribution.

Typical History

Tarsal tunnel syndrome can be caused by a variety of factors that create compression or tractioning of the tibial nerve. These include space-occupying lesions, a crush or stretch injury, inflammation, and swelling of the sheathed tendons that also travel through the tarsal tunnel, chronic eversion or excessive pronation, and a sudden increase in high-impact activities such as running, volleyball, and dance. Patients with diabetes or hypothyroidism may be at greater risk for developing tarsal tunnel syndrome.

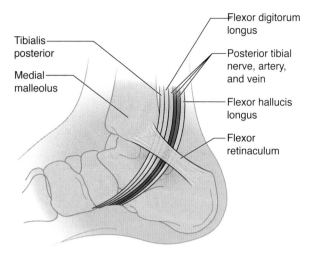

Tibialis posterior

Medial malleolus

Flexor digitorum longus

Posterior tibial nerve, artery, and vein

Flexor hallucis longus

Flexor retinaculum

FIGURE 8.41 Tarsal tunnel.

Relevant Anatomy

The tarsal tunnel is the channel formed between the underlying bony structure of the foot, primarily the medial malleolus and the calcaneus, and the flexor retinaculum (laciniate ligament). The tunnel consists of four canals that carry the sheathed tendons of the tibialis posterior, flexor digitorum longus, and flexor hallucis longus (Tom, Dick, and Harry muscles), as well as the posterior tibial nerve and artery vein (see figure 8.41).

Assessment

A thorough evaluation helps to determine whether the presenting symptoms are likely to be caused by tibial nerve entrapment at the tarsal tunnel and guide the possible treatment options.

Observation

The athlete may exhibit a pes planus (flat) foot. Swelling may also be present at the ankle and into the foot.

ROM Assessment

The athlete may exhibit excessive pronation of the affected foot. Eversion of the foot and dorsiflexion with toe extension may be limited by pain.

Manual Resistive Tests

Resisted inversion (see figure 8.42a) and resisted toe flexion (see figure 8.42b), especially the big toe, may be weak or painful.

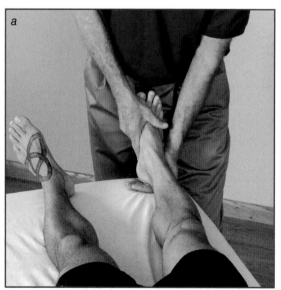
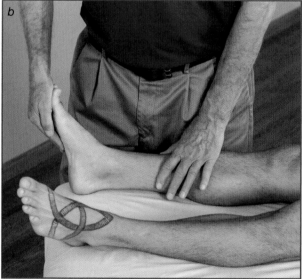

FIGURE 8.42 (a) Resisted inversion and (b) resisted toe flexion.

Nerve Glide Assessment

This assessment is used to evaluate the ability of the tibial nerve to move freely through the tarsal tunnel. Perform this assessment carefully to generate slight tension, but not to the point of discomfort. In this version of the nerve glide assessment, the athlete is supine on the treatment table with the legs straight. He slowly dorsiflexes the affected ankle to begin tensioning the tibial nerve (see figure 8.43a). If this position is comfortable, adding toe extension and ankle eversion will add more tension (see figure 8.43b). If at any point pain or paresthesia in the tibial nerve distribution is felt, the assessment is considered positive for tibial nerve involvement and stops.

Special Test

Tinel's test is commonly used to assess for tarsal tunnel syndrome as part of a thorough evaluation. The examiner dorsiflexes the ankle, everting the foot and extending the toes, then gently taps over the posterior tibial nerve at the tarsal tunnel (see figure 8.44). A positive test causes radiating pain and paresthesia along the nerve distribution into the foot and toes.

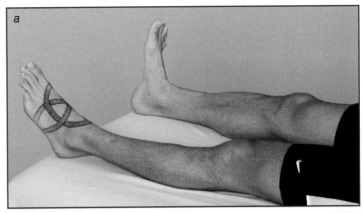

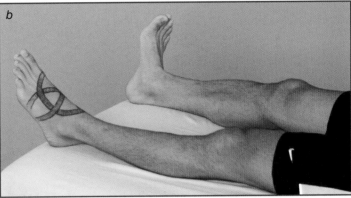

FIGURE 8.43 Tibial nerve glide assessment: *(a)* start with the ankle dorsiflexed and *(b)* add more tension to the tibial nerve by everting the ankle and extending the big toe.

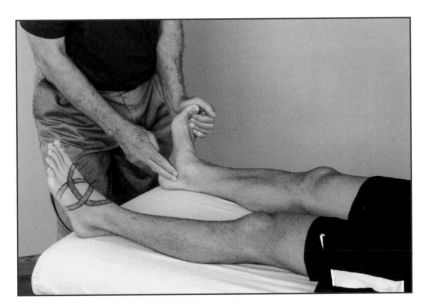

FIGURE 8.44 Tinel's test for tarsal tunnel syndrome.

Palpation

The palpatory exam around the medial ankle and plantar foot may reveal slight swelling or puffiness over the affected tissues and an increase in the athlete's symptoms.

Precautions and Contraindications

As with any nerve compression condition, additional compression or traction of the nerve that increases symptoms is to be avoided during treatment applications.

Differential Diagnosis

Plantar fasciitis, heel spurs, and retrocalcaneal bursitis.

Perpetuating Factors

Tarsal tunnel syndrome can be caused and perpetuated by many factors, including flat feet or chronic overpronation during walking, running, and jumping activities. Changing the pattern of use by reducing the frequency or intensity of the offending activities is critical during the healing process.

Treatment Plan

The overall goal for treatment is to reduce the compression on the tibial nerve and restore pain-free motion at the ankle and foot.

A typical treatment session is as follows:

1. Apply compressive effleurage and petrissage and broad cross-fiber work to the lower extremity as a general warm-up and to reduce the hypertonicity of the muscles, paying specific attention to the foot, ankle, and calf.

2. Administer facilitated stretching of the gastrocnemius, soleus, and toe flexors. Stretching that follows the warm-up massage helps further reduce hypertonicity and tension in the calf and foot.

3. Administer longitudinal stripping (see figure 8.45) and pin-and-stretch strokes (see figure 8.46) to the calf muscles.

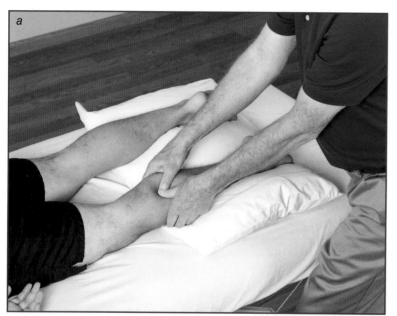

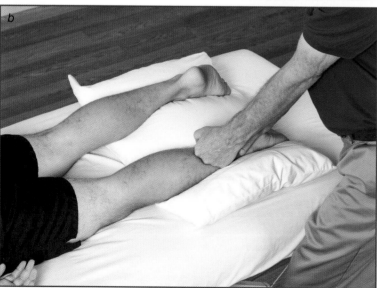

FIGURE 8.45   Longitudinal stripping of the calf muscles *(a)* with thumbs or *(b)* with a loose fist.

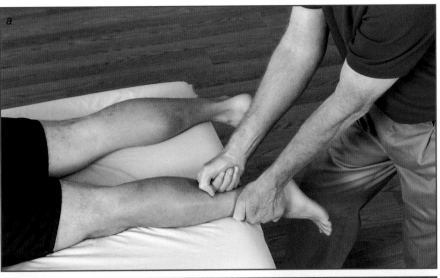

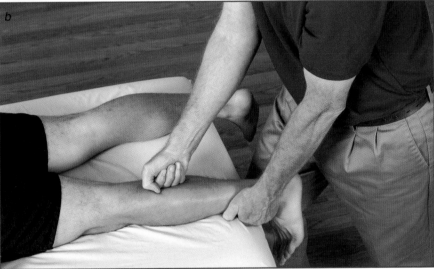

FIGURE 8.46   Pin and stretch of the calf muscles: *(a)* starting position with the ankle in plantar flexion to shorten the calf muscles and *(b)* ending position with the ankle fully dorsiflexed.

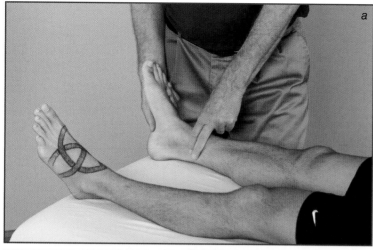

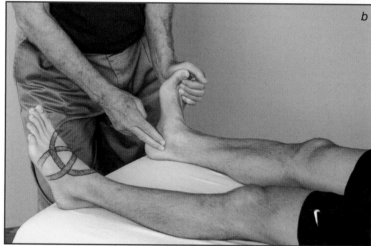

FIGURE 8.47 Transverse friction to *(a)* sheathed tendons near their myotendinous junctions and *(b)* as they course around the medial malleolus.

4. Use moderate-pressure general friction work to mobilize the tendons that pass through the tarsal tunnel. Use the fingers or thumb to apply moderate-pressure transverse friction to the tendons of the Tom, Dick, and Harry (TDH) muscles: tibialis posterior, flexor digitorum longus, and flexor hallucis longus at the medial ankle. These sheathed tendons are held on a slight stretch as friction is applied perpendicular to the tendon fibers (see figure 8.47).

5. Administer pain-free isolytic contractions to the calf muscles and toe flexors to help reduce protective inhibition and help the muscles return to full activation.

6. Finish the treatment with another round of facilitated stretching for the treated muscles.

Self-Care Options

If perpetuating factors are noted, these must be modified or eliminated to ensure that the injury does not reoccur. Once the symptoms have abated, initiate a program of flexibility and progressive strengthening. Focus on facilitated stretching for the gastrocnemius, soleus, toe flexors, and tibialis posterior, accompanied by strengthening exercise. Nerve glides help the nerve continue to move freely though the tarsal tunnel as it heals.

Piriformis syndrome (PS) is the name given to a complex of symptoms arising from compression of the sciatic nerve and associated blood vessels by the piriformis muscle as these structures exit the sciatic notch together. Two types of piriformis syndrome have been identified:

1. *Primary PS* is caused by an anatomical variation, such as an anomalous sciatic nerve path or a split sciatic nerve, in which part of the nerve passes through the piriformis muscle.

2. *Secondary PS* is the result of a precipitating cause, such as a macrotrauma, microtrauma, repetitive injury, altered biomechanics, or what is sometimes referred to as wallet neuritis.

Signs and Symptoms

The most common symptoms of piriformis syndrome are pain and paresthesia in the buttock and down the back of the leg. This pain generally originates at or below the sciatic notch, whereas in true sciatica, the pain originates at the lumbar spine (see figure 8.48).

Symptoms may be aggravated by prolonged sitting, by sitting with the affected leg crossed over the opposite knee, overstretching, or by activity such as running uphill or downhill, cycling in low gears, ballet and modern dance, and repetitive motions that overload the piriformis in its role as a stabilizer of the hip.

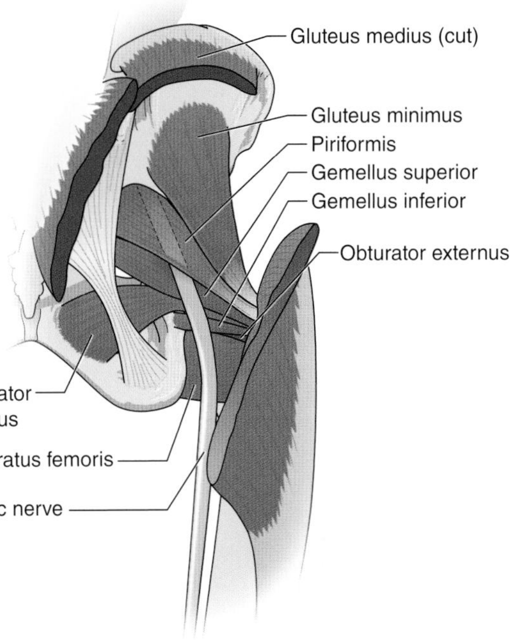

Typical History

Although traumatic piriformis syndrome may occur as the result of a fall or blow to the gluteal region, most cases develop slowly and are often the result of athletic activity or work-related tasks. Piriformis syndrome occurs most frequently during the fourth and fifth decades of life and affects people of all occupations and activity levels. Women are six times more likely than men to experience PS, possibly because of the biomechanics associated with the wider Q angle in the female pelvis.

FIGURE 8.48 Piriformis syndrome symptoms usually begin at or below the sciatic notch, not at the lumbar spine.

Both vascular and nerve entrapment occur primarily at the greater sciatic foramen. In some cases, the piriformis muscle is hypertrophic and leaves little room for free passage of the sciatic nerve and associated blood vessels. In other cases, chronic hypertonicity that makes the piriformis short and thick is sufficient to fill the foramen and compress the nerve. In addition, anatomic anomalies may predispose an athlete to develop this condition. According to Muscolino (2017, para 2), "approximately 10% to 20% of the time, part or all of the sciatic nerve either exits through the piriformis, or above it, between the piriformis and the gluteus medius."

Sacroiliac (SI) joint dysfunction is also a likely component of piriformis syndrome. Because of the location of its origin on the anterior sacrum, the piriformis can produce a rotary shearing force on the SI joint, which would tend to displace the top of the sacrum anteriorly. This may translate into an anterior tilt of the

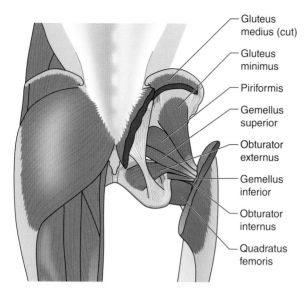

FIGURE 8.49 The piriformis is one of the lateral rotators of the hip.
© Human Kinetics

posterior superior iliac spine (PSIS) when compared to the opposite side. Manipulation of the SI joint without resolving piriformis hypertonicity will give only brief relief. Likewise, attempting to relieve piriformis hypertonicity without addressing the SI joint displacement is ineffective.

Relevant Anatomy

The piriformis is one of the deep-six lateral rotators and the muscle most often the culprit in piriformis syndrome (see figure 8.49). Sciatic nerve entrapment in the gluteal region can also occur at the quadratus femoris muscle. The piriformis originates from the anterior sacrum, between and lateral to the first through the fourth sacral foramina, sometimes receiving additional fibers from the sacrotuberous and sacrospinous ligaments and the upper margin of the sciatic notch at the capsule of the sacroiliac joint. The piriformis inserts into the medial side of the superior aspect of the greater trochanter. The tendon may blend with the tendons of the obturator internus and the gemelli inferior and superior.

The piriformis, along with the gemelli, the obturators, and the quadratus femoris laterally rotates the femur. However, the degree of hip flexion affects the action of the piriformis muscle. At 90° of hip flexion, the piriformis becomes a horizontal abductor of the femur, and with full hip flexion, the piriformis medially rotates the femur, reversing its action as a lateral rotator. The piriformis also acts as a stabilizer of the hip and, along with the other lateral rotators, helps hold the femoral head within the acetabulum, forming a rotator cuff for the hip, and acts eccentrically to control medial rotation of the thigh in walking and running.

Assessment

Investigation of this condition can be challenging because the symptoms of piriformis syndrome are also consistent with the symptoms of lumbar radiculopathy and trochanteric bursitis.

Observation

With the client standing relaxed in bare feet, check for level iliac crests, PSIS, and anterior superior iliac spine (ASIS). Also note whether one PSIS is anterior compared to the other. Imbalance in these areas is common in piriformis syndrome.

Morton's foot and overpronation cause excessive medial rotation and adduction of the thigh during running and walking, overworking the piriformis eccentrically as it attempts to counteract medial rotation. This may lead to hypertonicity. With the patient supine on the treatment table, compare lateral rotation of the hips (see figure 8.50). Excessive lateral rotation (45° or more) indicates piriformis shortening on that side. This becomes relevant if the excessive rotation is on the symptomatic side.

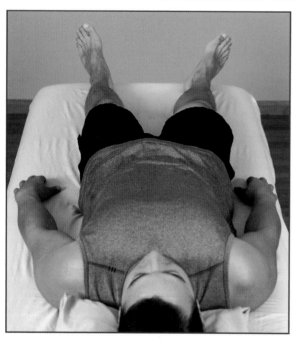

FIGURE 8.50 Compare lateral rotation of the femurs. This athlete exhibits excessive lateral rotation on the right, which may indicate hypertonicity in the lateral rotators. This finding is relevant if it occurs on the symptomatic side.

ROM Assessment

Assess for ROM in lateral and medial rotation in the prone position (see figure 8.51). Normal range for lateral rotation is 45°, and normal range for medial rotation is 35° to 45°.

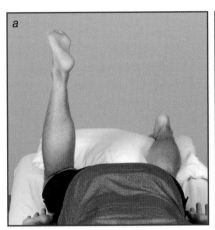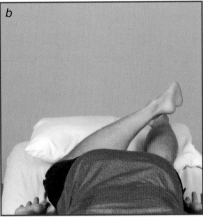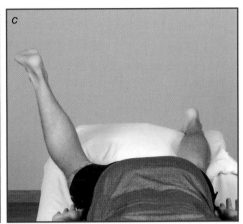

FIGURE 8.51   Assess for normal ROM in hip rotation. Lateral rotation is typically about 45° and medial rotation usually falls between 35° to 45°.

Manual Resistive Testing

Assessment of the piriformis can include several tests that isolate the muscle. Once a positive finding has been made, further testing is not needed.

Pace Abduction Test

The Pace test is a manual resisted assessment and may put stress on the sciatic nerve as the piriformis muscle contracts as an abductor in this position. This test is thought to be more effective than resisted lateral rotation of the hip because it eliminates the other five lateral rotators. With the client seated with knees flexed and hanging over the edge of the table, the examiner places his hands on the lateral knees and directs the client to slowly attempt to push the legs apart as the examiner provides matching resistance to prevent movement (resisted abduction) (see figure 8.52). If this elicits no pain, the client pushes harder until maximal effort is achieved. On the other hand, if pain, faltering, or weakness occurs, the test is considered positive for piriformis involvement, and the test is concluded.

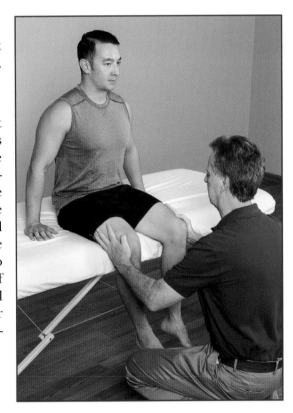

FIGURE 8.52   The Pace abduction test is an isometric test of hip abduction that may stress the sciatic nerve.

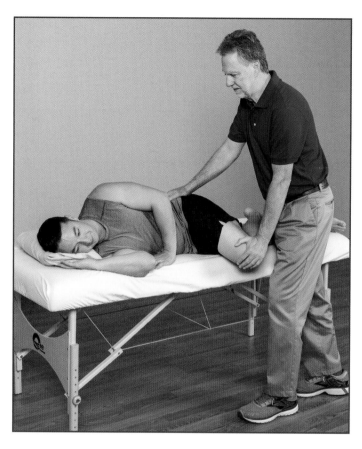

FAIR Test

The FAIR test (flexion, adduction, and internal rotation) is a passive assessment that stretches the piriformis and may compress the sciatic nerve against the underlying bone. The client lies on the unaffected side, the hips stacked vertically, the bottom leg straight, and the top hip and knee flexed to approximately 90°, with the foot tucked behind the bottom knee if possible. The client is positioned near the edge of the table so the knee of the test leg can drop over the side. From this starting position, the examiner stabilizes the hips with one hand and passively adducts and internally rotates the test leg (pressing the knee toward the floor) (see figure 8.53). Painful limitation of adduction is positive for piriformis involvement.

FIGURE 8.53 The FAIR test passively stretches piriformis and may compress the sciatic nerve.

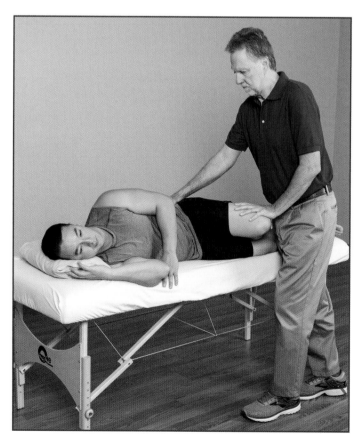

Beatty Maneuver

The Beatty maneuver is a manual resisted assessment and may put stress on the sciatic nerve as the muscle contracts. This is conducted the same as the Pace test, but from a side-lying position. The client lies on the unaffected side, the hips stacked vertically, the bottom leg straight, and the top hip and knee flexed to approximately 90°, with the foot tucked behind the bottom knee if possible. Instead of passive adduction as in the FAIR test, the client attempts to press the knee toward the ceiling as the examiner provides matching resistance to prevent movement (resisted abduction) (see figure 8.54). If there is no pain, the client pushes harder until maximal effort is achieved. On the other hand, if pain, faltering, or weakness occurs, the test is considered positive for piriformis involvement, and the test is concluded.

FIGURE 8.54 The Beatty maneuver is a resisted abduction test of the piriformis that may compress the sciatic nerve.

Palpation

The piriformis lies deep to the gluteus maximus, which must remain relaxed during the palpatory exam. To accurately locate the piriformis, identify the bony landmarks of the superior greater trochanter (the insertion) and the greater sciatic foramen, adjacent to the lateral sacrum, where the piriformis emerges from its origin on the anterior sacrum.

The piriformis muscle is palpated superior to the level of its insertion into the greater trochanter. Palpation along the length and across the grain of the muscle may reveal taut bands, trigger points, tenderness, and "nervy" pain. Taut bands and tenderness inferior to the piriformis are most likely located in the gemelli, obturator internus, and quadratus femoris. If palpation elicits nerve pain, the practitioner moves the palpatory contact slightly, away from the sciatic nerve and checks to see whether the quality of pain changes. To avoid contacting the sciatic nerve, use caution when palpating at the greater sciatic foramen and at a point halfway between the ischial tuberosity and the greater trochanter as the nerve passes over the quadratus femoris and into the leg.

Precautions and Contraindications

Care must be taken when palpating for and treating nerve compression syndromes to avoid further irritation of already compromised neural structures.

Differential Diagnosis

Degenerative lumbar disc, spinal stenosis, trochanteric bursitis, and sacroiliac joint dysfunction.

Perpetuating Factors

Training factors that lead to and perpetuate piriformis syndrome are hill running, speed work, excessive time spent in lateral rotation (as in ballet), and stop and start sports (such as tennis, racquetball, volleyball, soccer). Biomechanical factors contributing to piriformis syndrome include SI joint dysfunction, Morton's foot, overpronation, leg-length difference, and weak medial rotators. Equipment-related factors include worn or improperly fitting running shoes or long periods of sitting with pressure on the piriformis during activities such as computer work and driving.

Treatment Plan

Piriformis syndrome is primarily a nerve compression condition. Treatment must be aimed at relieving the pressure on the nerve. Deep transverse friction is not usually applicable in this case. Massage and stretching to relieve hypertonicity of the gluteal muscles and all of the lateral rotators of the hip will be the most effective treatment.

A typical treatment session is as follows:

1. Apply compressive effleurage and petrissage and broad cross-fiber work to the gluteal region as a general warm-up and to reduce the hypertonicity of the muscles, paying specific attention to the gluteus maximus and medius.

2. Administer facilitated stretching of the lateral rotator muscle group. Stretching that follows the warm-up massage helps further reduce hypertonicity and tension in the posterior hip muscles.

3. Apply pain-free transverse friction to the attachments along the entire sacral border. Treatment of the posterior ilium and the piriformis insertion on the greater trochanter is especially effective when the piriformis has been warmed up with other techniques (see figure 8.55).

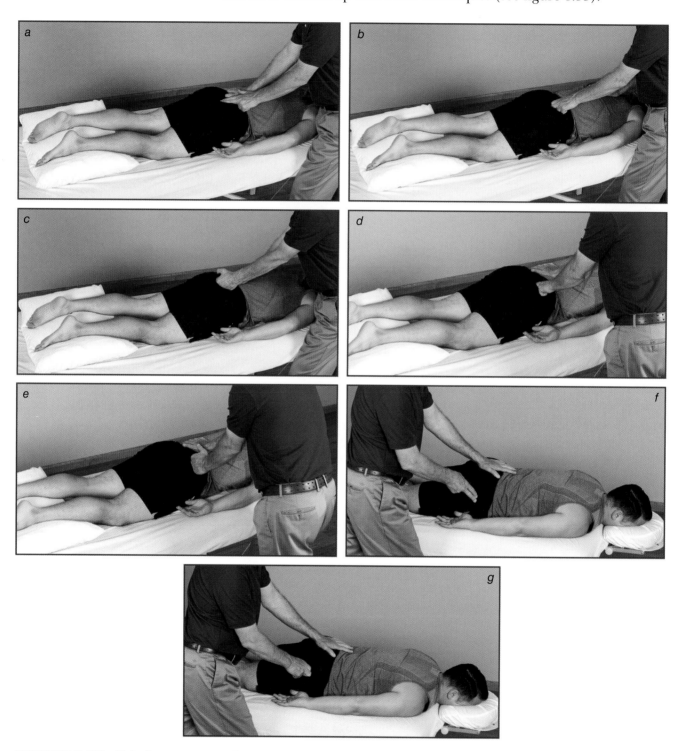

FIGURE 8.55 Pain-free transverse friction to the sacral border with *(a)* flat fingers or *(b)* flat knuckles or *(c)* loose fist, to the posterior ilium with *(d)* flat knuckles or *(e)* a loose fist, and around the greater trochanter with *(f)* flat fingers or *(g)* flat knuckles.

4. Administer pain-free pin and stretch through the entire gluteal region (see figure 8.56). The first pass is performed with a broad contact (e.g., a loose fist). On the second pass, a narrower contact is used (e.g., a flat thumb or soft knuckles). During the second and subsequent passes, careful attention is directed toward specific areas of fibrosity or hypertonicity.

5. Administer pain-free isolytic contractions to the lateral rotators to help reduce protective inhibition and help the muscles return to full activation (see figure 8.57). Stabilize the hips at the sacrum and avoid pressing into the piriformis while it's contracting.

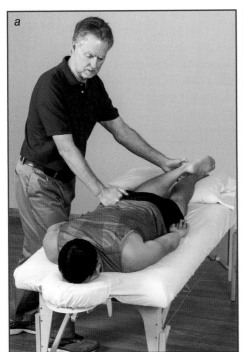
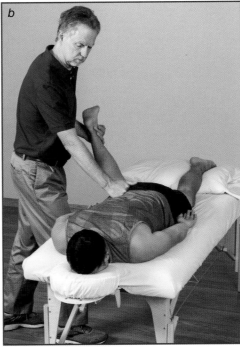

FIGURE 8.56 Pin and stretch of the piriformis with a loose fist: *(a)* starting position with the piriformis passively shortened and pinned and *(b)* maintaining the pin pressure to the ending position with the piriformis fully lengthened.

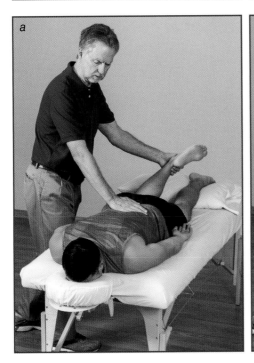
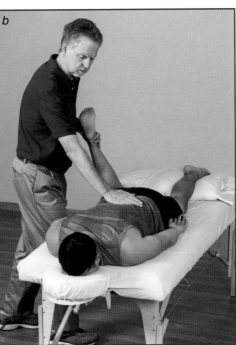

FIGURE 8.57 Isolytic contractions for the piriformis: *(a)* starting position with one hand stabilizing the hips at the sacrum and the other hand used to rotate the femur, lengthening the piriformis, while the athlete is resisting at the appropriate level of effort; and *(b)* the ending position with the piriformis fully lengthened.

6. Finish the treatment with another round of facilitated stretching for the treated muscles.

Self-Care Options

If perpetuating factors are noted, these must be modified or eliminated to ensure that the injury does not reoccur. Once the symptoms have abated, initiate a program of flexibility and progressive strengthening. Focus on facilitated stretching for the lateral rotator group and the gluteus medius. Strengthening work can begin after biomechanical imbalances are corrected.

APPENDIX A

Research Resources

American Massage Therapy Association website (Research Roundups): www. amtamassage.org/research/Massage-Therapy-Research-Roundup.html

Association of Massage Therapists (Australia) website (Research database): www. amt.org.au/members/research-resources.html

Evidence-Informed Massage Therapy Facebook Page: www.facebook.com/massage. evidence

International Journal of Therapeutic Massage and Bodywork: www.ijtmb.org

Massage Magazine (Research Studies section): www.massagemag.com/ research-studies

Massage Therapy Canada website (Research section): www.massagetherapycanada. com/research

Massage Therapy Foundation: www.massagetherapyfoundation.org

REFERENCES

Alomar AZ. Groin pain in athletes: differential diagnosis, assessment, and management. *Saudi Journal of Sports Medicine.* 2015; 15 (1): 3–8.

Archer P. *Therapeutic massage in athletics.* Baltimore, MD: Lippincott Williams & Wilkins; 2007.

Ashworth NL. Carpal tunnel syndrome clinical presentation. [revised 2018 Feb 27; cited 2018 May 12] Available from: https://emedicine.medscape.com/article/327330-clinical\

Ballal MS, Walker CR, Molloy AP. The anatomical footprint of the Achilles tendon, a cadaveric study. *The Bone & Joint Journal* 2014; 96-B (10): 1344–1348. doi: 10.1302/0301-620X.96B10.33771.

Bass E. Tendinopathy: why the difference between tendinitis and tendinosis matters. *Int J Ther Massage Bodywork.* 2012; 5 (1): 14–17.

Bisio TA. Tooth from the tiger's mouth. New York, NY: Simon and Schuster; 2004.

Bleakley CM, Glasgow P, MacAuley DC. PRICE needs updating, should we call the POLICE? *Br J Sports Med.* 2012 Mar; 46 (4): 220–221.

Bleakley C, McDonough S, MacAuley DC. The use of ice in the treatment of acute soft-tissue injury. *Am J Sports Med.* 2004 Jan-Feb; 32 (1): 251–261.

Brown S, Doolittle DA, Bohanon CJ, Jayaraj A, Naidu SG, Huettl EA, et al. Quadrilateral space syndrome. *Mayo Clin Proc.* 2015 Mar; 90 (3): 382–394.

Buckwalter JA. Activity vs. rest in the treatment of bone, soft tissue and joint injuries. *The Iowa Orthopaedic Journal.* 1995; 15: 29–42.

Butler DS. The sensitive nervous system. Adelaide, Australia: Noigroup Publications; 2000.

Butterfield, TA, Zhao Y, Agarwal S, Haq F, Best T. Cyclic compressive loading facilitates recovery after eccentric exercise. *Med Sci Sports and Exerc.* 2008 Jul; 40 (7): 1289–1296.

Chaitow L. Muscle energy techniques. 2nd ed. London, UK: Churchill Livingstone; 2001.

Chaitow L. We have much to learn from current fascia research. 2016 Sep 18 [cited 2018 Aug 1] Available from http://leonchaitow.com/2016/09/18/we-have-much-to-learn-from-current-fascia-research/.

Churgay CA. Diagnosis and treatment of biceps tendinitis and tendinosis. *Am Fam Physician.* 2009 Sep 1; 80 (5): 470–476.

Clement DB, Taunton JE, Smart GW. Achilles tendinitis and peritendinitis: etiology and treatment. *Am J Sports Med.* 1984 May-Jun; 12 (3): 179–184.

Crane JD, Ogborn DI, Cupido1 C, Melov S, Hubbard A, Bourgeois JM, et al. Massage therapy attenuates inflammatory signaling after exercise-induced muscle damage. *Sci Transl Med.* 2012 Feb 1; 4 (119): 119ra13. doi:10.1126/scitranslmed.3002882.

Cushman D, Rho M. Conservative treatment of subacute proximal hamstring tendinopathy using eccentric exercises performed with a treadmill: a case report. *J Orthop Sports Phys Ther.* 2015 Jul; 45 (7): 557–562.

Cutts S. Cubital tunnel syndrome. *Postgrad Med J.* 2007 Jan; 83 (975): 28–31. doi:10.1136/pgmj.2006.047456.

Cyriax J, Cyriax P. *Cyriax's illustrated manual of orthopaedic medicine.* London, UK: Butterworths; 1983.

Duke University Web Tutorial [Internet]. Introduction to evidence-based practice. [revised 2014 December; cited 2018 Sep 24]. Available from: https://guides. mclibrary.duke.edu/c.php?g=158201&p=1036021.

Duncan R. *Myofascial release: hands-on guides for therapists.* Champaign, IL: Human Kinetics; 2014.

Edama M, Kubo M, Onishi H, Takabayashi T, Inai T, Yokoyama E, et al. The twisted structure of the human Achilles tendon. *Scand J Med Sci Sports.* 2015 Oct; 25: e497–e503. doi:10.1111/sms.12342.

Elliott R, Burkett B. Massage therapy as an effective treatment for carpal tunnel syndrome. *J Bodyw Mov Ther.* 2013 Jul; 17 (3): 332–338. doi:10.1016/j. jbmt.2012.12.003.

Elvey R. *The investigation of arm pain. Grieve's modern manual therapy: the vertebral column.* 2nd ed. Boyling JD, Palastanga N, editors. Edinburgh, UK: Churchill Livingstone; 1994.

Enoka, R. *Neuromechanics of human movement.* 5th ed. Champaign, IL: Human Kinetics; 2015.

Fairbank SM, Corlett RJ. *The role of the extensor digitorum communis muscle in lateral epicondylitis. J Hand Surg Br.* 2002 Oct; 27 (5): 405–409.

Fairclough J, Hayashi K, Toumi H, Lyons K, Bydder G, Phillips N, et al. Is ITB syndrome really a friction syndrome? *J Sci Med Sport.* 2007 Apr; 10 (2): 74–76.

Field T, Diego M, Cullen C, Hartshorn K, Gruskin A, Hernandez-Reif M, et al. Carpal tunnel syndrome symptoms are lessened following massage therapy. *J Bodyw Mov. Ther.* 2004; 8 (1): 9–14.

Field T, Diego M, Hernandez-Reif M. Moderate pressure is essential for massage therapy effects. *Int J Neurosci.* 2010 May; 120 (5): 381–385.

Finch PM. The evidence funnel: highlighting the importance of research literacy in the delivery of evidence informed complementary health care. *J. Bodyw. Mov. Ther.* 2007; 11 (1): 78–81.

Fritz S. *Sports and exercise massage.* 2nd ed. St. Louis, MO: Elsevier Mosby; 2013.

Funk L. Quadrilateral space syndrome. Shoulderdoc.co.uk. n.d. [cited 2018 Feb 24]. Available from: https://www.shoulderdoc.co.uk/article/1366.

Garg K, Corona BT, Walters TJ. Therapeutic strategies for preventing skeletal muscle fibrosis after injury. *Front Pharmacol.* 2015 Apr 21; 6: 87. doi:10.3389/ fphar.2015.00087.

Geisler P, Lazenby T. An evidence-informed clinical paradigm change. *International Journal of Athletic Training & Therapy.* 2017; 22 (3): 1–11.

Gleason PD, Beall DP, Sanders TG, Bond JL, Ly JQ, Holland LL. The transverse humeral ligament: a separate anatomical structure or a continuation of the osseous attachment of the rotator cuff? *Am J Sports Med.* 2006 Jan; 34 (1): 72–77. Epub 2005 Sep 16.

Hanna AS, Fried TB, Ghobrial GM, Harrop JS, Spinner RJ, Nosko MG. Nerve entrapment syndromes. 2017 Sep 21 [cited 2018 Nov 3] Available from: https://emedicine.medscape.com/article/24978.

Harris J, Kenyon F. *Fix pain: bodywork protocols for myofascial pain syndromes.* Santa Barbara, CA: Press4Health; 2002.

Ingraham, P. Deep friction massage therapy for tendinitis. 2018a [revised 2018 March; cited 2018 Jul 17]. Available from: https://www.painscience.com/articles/frictions.php.

Ingraham, P. Save yourself from IT band syndrome! 2018b [revised 2018 Sep 22; cited 2018 Oct 21]. Available from: https://www.painscience.com/tutorials/iliotibial-band-syndrome.php.

Jurch, S. Pulling back the curtain: a look at sports massage therapy. 2015. American Massage Therapy Association [Internet]. [cited 2018 Feb 24] Available from: www.amtamassage.org/uploads/cms/documents/sports_jurch.pdf.

Kerkhoffs GM, Rowe BH, Assendelft WJ, Kelly K, Struijs PA, van Dijk CN. Immobilisation and functional treatment for acute lateral ankle ligament injuries in adults. *Cochrane Database Syst Rev.* 2002; (3): CD003762.

Kim J, Sung DJ, Lee J. Therapeutic effectiveness of instrument-assisted soft tissue mobilization for soft tissue injury: mechanisms and practical application. *J Exerc Rehabil.* 2017 Feb; 13 (1): 12–22. doi:10.12965/jer.1732824.412.

King R. *Performance massage.* Champaign, IL: Human Kinetics; 1993.

Kohn HS. Prevention and treatment of elbow injuries in golf. *Clin Sports Med.* 1996 Jan; 15 (1): 65–83.

Kumai T, Takakura Y, Rufai A, Milz S, Benjamin M. The functional anatomy of the human anterior talofibular ligament in relation to ankle sprains. *J Anat.* 2002 May; 200 (5): 457–465.

Lemont H, Ammirati KM, Usen N. Plantar fasciitis: a degenerative process (fasciosis) without inflammation. *J Am Podiatr Med Assoc.* 2003 May-Jun; 93 (3): 234–237.

Li H-Y, Hua Y-H. Achilles tendinopathy: current concepts about the basic science and clinical treatments. *BioMed Research International.* 2016: 6492597. doi:10.1155/2016/6492597.

Lohrer H, Nauck T, Arentz S, Vogl TJ. Dorsal calcaneocuboid ligament versus lateral ankle ligament repair: a case-control study. *Br J Sports Med.* 2006 Oct; 40 (10): 839–843.

Lowe W. Maybe that's not tennis elbow. *Massage Today.* 2015 Nov; 15 (11). [cited 2018 Jul 17] Available from: https://www.massagetoday.com/mpacms/mt/article.php?id=15125.

Lowe W. Deciphering elusive symptoms of nerve injury. 2018 Jan 17 [cited 2018 Sep 24] Available from: https://www.academyofclinicalmassage.com/deciphering-elusive-symptoms-nerve-injury.

Lowe W. Exploring upper limb neurodynamics. 2016 Jul 14 [cited 2018 Sep 24] Available from: thttps://www.academyofclinicalmassage.com/exploring-upper-limb-neurodynamics.

Lowe W. Confronting the challenges of a major paradigm shift. 2017 Sep 28 [cited 2018 Sep 24] Available from: https://www.academyofclinicalmassage.com/confronting-challenges-major-paradigm-shift/.

Maas H, Sandercock TG. Force transmission between synergistic skeletal muscles through connective tissue linkages. *J Biomed Biotechno.* 2010. doi: 10.1155/2010/575672.

Mann CJ, Perdiguero E, Kharraz, Y, Auguilar S, Pessina P, Serrano AL, et al. Aberrant repair and fibrosis development in skeletal muscle. *Skeletal Muscle*, 2011 May 4; 1 (1): 21.

Mattingly G, Mackarey P. Optimal methods for shoulder tendon palpation: a cadaver study. *Phys Ther.* 1996 Feb; 76 (2): 166–173.

McAtee R, Charland J. *Facilitated stretching.* 4th ed. Champaign, IL: Human Kinetics; 2014.

Mirkin G. Why ice delays recovery. drmirkin.com. 2015 [cited 2018 May 3] Available from: www.drmirkin.com/fitness/why-ice-delays-recovery.html.

Mirkin G, Hoffman M. *The Sports Medicine Book.* Boston, MA: Little, Brown & Co; 1978

Muscolino J. Piriformis syndrome. Learnmuscles.com 2017. [cited 2018 Sep 22] Available from: https://learnmuscles.com/blog/2017/09/05/piriformis-syndrome/

Ooi SL, Smith L, Pak SC. Evidence-informed massage therapy – an Australian practitioner perspective. *Complement Ther Clin Pract.* 2018 May; 31: 325–331.

Orchard J, Best TM. The management of muscle strain injuries: an early return versus the risk of recurrence. *Clin J Sport Med.* 2002 Jan; 12 (1): 3–5.

Parmar S, Shyam A, Sabnis S, Sancheti P. The effect of isolytic contraction and passive manual stretching on pain and knee range of motion after hip surgery: a prospective, double-blinded, randomized study. *Hong Kong Physiotherapy Journal.* 2011; 29 (1): 25–30.

Pękala PA, Henry BM, Ochała A, Kopacz P, Taton G, Mlyniec A, Walocha JA, Tomaszewski KA. The twisted structure of the Achilles tendon unraveled: A detailed quantitative and qualitative anatomical investigation. *Scand J Med Sci Sports.* 2017; 27: 1705–1715. https://doi.org/10.1111/sms.12835.

Rather LJ. Disturbance of function (functio laesa): the legendary fifth cardinal sign of inflammation, added by Galen to the four cardinal signs of Celsus. *Bull N Y Acad Med.* 1971 Mar; 47 (3): 303–322.

Rees JD, Stride M, Scott A. Tendons – time to revisit inflammation. *Br J Sports Med.* 2014 Nov; 48 (21): 1553–1557. doi:10.1136/bjsports-2012-091957.

Reinl, G. *Iced: the illusionary treatment option.* 2nd ed. Henderson, NV: Gary Reinl; 2014.

Rio E, Kidgell D, Purdam C, Gaida J, Moseley GL, Parce AJ, et al. Isometric exercise induces analgesia and reduces inhibition in patellar tendinopathy. *Br J Sports Med.* 2015 Oct; 49: 1277–1283.

Rudavsky A, Cook J. Physiotherapy management of patellar tendinopathy (jumper's knee). *J Physiother.* 2014 Sep; 60 (3): 122–129.

Sanders RJ, Hammond SL, Rao NM. Diagnosis of thoracic outlet syndrome. *J Vasc Surg.* 2007 Sep; 46 (3): 601–604.

Shibaguchi T, Sugiura T, Fujitsu T, Nomura T, Yoshihara T, Naito H, Yoshioka T, Ogura A, Ohira Y. Effects of icing or heat stress on the induction of fibrosis and/or regeneration of injured rat soleus muscle. *J Physiol Sci.* 2016 Jul; 66 (4): 345–357.

Shultz SJ, Houglum PA, Perring DH. *Examination of musculoskeletal injuries.* 2nd ed. Champaign, IL: Human Kinetics; 2005.

Shurygina EV. Function of scalene muscles under conditions of quiet breathing and inspiratory resistive load. *Bull Exp Biol Med.* 1999 Dec; 128 (6): 1199–1202.

Smith LL, Keating MN, Holbert D, Spratt DJ, McCammon MR, Smith SS, et al. The effects of athletic massage on delayed onset muscle soreness, creatine kinase, and neutrophil count: a preliminary report. *J Orthop Sports Phys Ther.* 1994 Feb; 19 (2): 93–99.

Stecco C, Corradin M, Macchi V, Morra A, Porzionato A, Biz C, et al. Plantar fascia anatomy and its relationship with Achilles tendon and paratenon. *J Anat.* 2013 Dec; 223 (6): 665–676. doi:10.1111/joa.12111.

Stecco C. *Functional atlas of the human fascial system.* London, UK: Churchill Livingstone/Elsevier; 2015.

Stone, J. *Icing injuries: are we evidence based?* 2014 Sep 20 [cited 2018 May 3] Available from: http://stoneathleticmedicine.com/2014/09/icing-injuries-are-we-evidence-based/.

Tahririan MA, Motififard M, Tahmasebi MN, Siavashi B. Plantar fasciitis. *Journal of Research in Medical Sciences: The Official Journal of Isfahan University of Medical Sciences.* 2012; 17 (8): 799–804.

Takagi R, Fujita N, Arakawa T, Kawada S, Ishii N, Miki A. Influence of icing on muscle regeneration after crush injury to skeletal muscles in rats. *J of App Phys.* 2011 Feb; 110 (2): 382–388.

Travell JG, Simons DG. *Myofascial pain and dysfunction: the trigger point manual.* vol. 2. Philadelphia, PA: Williams and Wilkins; 1992.

Tyler TF, Campbell R, Nicholas SJ, Donellan S, McHugh MP. The effectiveness of a preseason exercise program on the prevention of groin strains in professional ice hockey players. *Am J Sports Med.* 2002 Sep-Oct; 30 (5): 680–683.

Tyler TF, Silvers HJ, Gerhardt MB, Nicholas SJ. Groin injuries in sports medicine. *Sports Health.* 2010 May; 2 (3): 231–236.

van der Wal, J. The architecture of the connective tissue in the musculoskeletal system—an often overlooked functional parameter as to proprioception in the locomotor apparatus. *Int J Ther Massage Bodywork.* 2009 Dec 7; 2 (4): 9–23.

Van Sterkenburg MN, van Dijk CN. Mid-portion Achilles tendinopathy: why painful? An evidence-based philosophy. *Knee Surgery, Sports Traumatology, Arthroscopy.* 2011; 19 (8): 1367–1375. doi:10.1007/s00167-011-1535-8.

Waters-Banker C, Dupont-Versteegden EE, Kitzman PH, Butterfield TA. Investigating the mechanisms of massage efficacy: the role of mechanical immunomodulation. *J Athl Train.* 2014 Mar-Apr; 49 (2): 266–273. doi:10.4085/1062-6050-49.2.25.

Willard FH, Vleeming A, Schuenke MD, Danneels L, Schleip R. The thoracolumbar fascia: anatomy, function and clinical considerations. *J Anat.* 2012 Dec; 221 (6): 507–536. doi:10.1111/j.1469-7580.2012.01511.x.

Zitnay JL, Li Y, Qin Z, San BH, Depalle B, Reese SP, et al. Molecular level detection and localization of mechanical damage in collagen enabled by collagen hybridizing peptides. *Nat. Commun.* 2017 Mar 22; 8: 14913. doi:10.1038/ncomms14913.

INDEX

Note: The italicized *f* and *t* following page numbers refer to figures and tables, respectively.

ABOUT THE AUTHOR

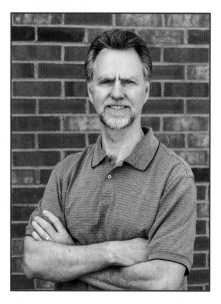

Robert E. McAtee, BA, LMT, BCTMB, CSCS, has maintained a full-time massage therapy practice for over 38 years, specializing in sports massage and soft tissue therapy, with significant clinical experience in treating people with injuries and chronic pain. Since 1988, he has owned Pro-Active Massage Therapy, an international private practice in Colorado Springs, Colorado.

McAtee is designated an Approved Provider by the National Certification Board for Therapeutic Massage and Bodywork (NCBTMB). He is a sought-after presenter—throughout the United States and worldwide—on the topics of facilitated stretching, sports massage, and soft tissue injury care.

McAtee received his massage training at the Institute for Psycho-Structural Balancing (IPSB) in Los Angeles and San Diego and through the Sports Massage Training Institute (SMTI) in Costa Mesa, California. He holds a bachelor's degree in psychology from California State University, is board certified in therapeutic massage and bodywork, and is a certified strength and conditioning specialist. He has been an active member of the American Massage Therapy Association since 1988.

He is also the coauthor of the best-selling book *Facilitated Stretching*, Fourth Edition, used by health and fitness professionals worldwide as their go-to resource for PNF stretching and strengthening techniques.

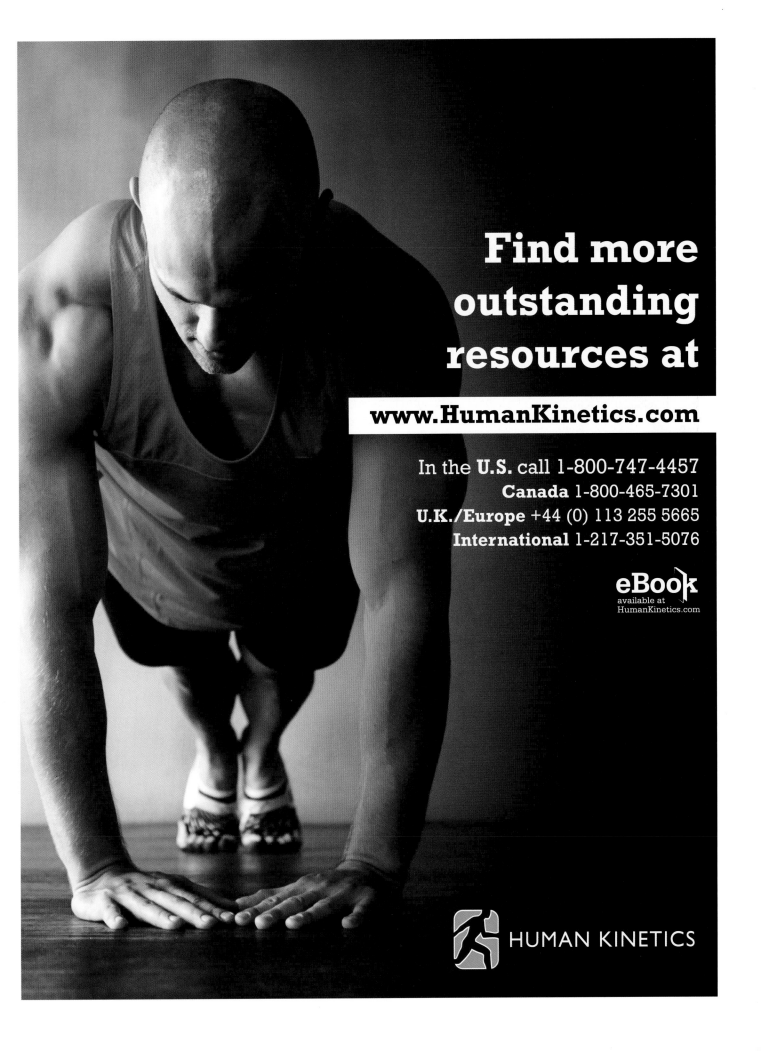

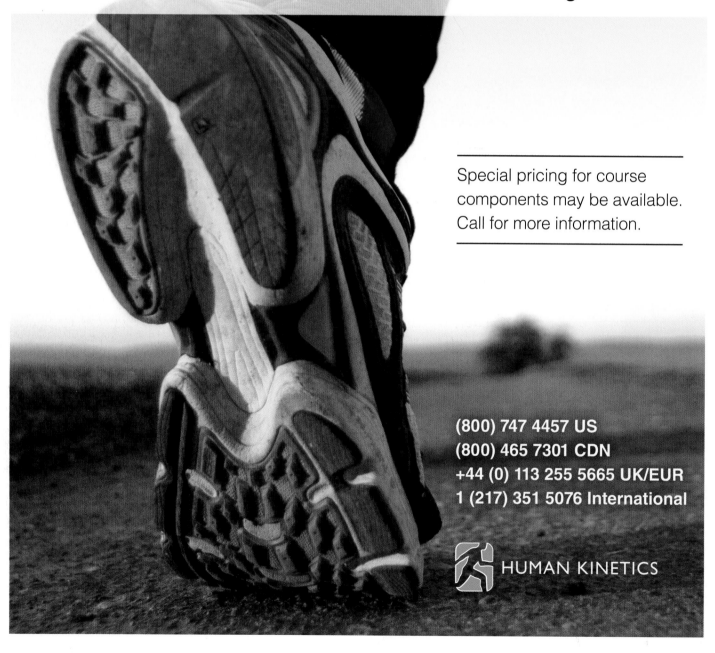